Beyond Psychotherapy

Introduction to Psychoenergetic Healing

by

Martin F. Luthke, Ph.D.
&
Linda Stein-Luthke

Expansion Publishing

Beyond Psychotherapy

Introduction to Psychoenergetic Healing

First printing: 2001

ISBN 0-9656927-4-4

Cover design by Dennis Sutton, Studio East, Akron, OH
<dennis@studioeast.com>

Manufactured in the USA by Publishers' Graphics, Nashville, TN.

Published by

Expansion Publishing
P.O. Box 516 - Chagrin Falls, OH 44022
USA

Contents

Acknowledgments

We would like to thank

- Our editor, Julianne Stein, for her loving dedication
- Our clients, for the many gifts we have received through working with them
- The Ascended Masters, for their patience, guidance, and Love
- Our cats, Samuel and Lucky, for their unique contributions to the manuscript.

Introduction

About the Authors

Martin Luthke: I am the one who put this material on paper. However, without the inspiration, insights, guidance, and contributions of my wife, the body of knowledge contained in this book never would have developed. Thus, Linda rightfully deserves the title of co-author.

I was born in 1956 in Bremen, Germany. My professional biography includes training as a cabinetmaker and carpenter, three semesters of medical school (which I decided to leave for lack of fun), and a Ph.D. in psychology from the University of Hamburg. In 1987 I came to the USA to attend a Ph.D.-program in clinical psychology at the University of Cincinnati. I completed the program plus internships and received a Certificate of Respecialization in clinical psychology.

After practicing as a child and adolescent psychologist at a child guidance center for some time, I decided to develop my own work in the relative freedom of independent practice. Perpetually searching for better tools, I pursued training in psychodrama, hypnosis, Thought Field Therapy, Emotional Freedom Techniques, Hypno-Kinesiology, Reiki, Polarity, Reflexology, and Swedish massage.

Beginning in my youth, I studied the literature of psychoanalysis, a school of thought that held my interest for a long time. (At one point I even applied for training as a psychoanalyst.) My academic training spans a total of 14 years spent at universities, studying, researching, teaching, and writing a dozen publications. I received excellent grades and several stipends and scholarships, and I passed the national licensure exam in the top one percent. All this I mention solely to indicate that I *did* put more than my share of time and effort into learning the tools of my trade -- and yet my path took me away from the "conventional wisdom" currently accepted and taught in the fields of healing and psychotherapy.

Linda Stein-Luthke is a writer, astrologer, metaphysical teacher, and healer with exceptional intuitive abilities. She has raised two sons (and cared for two foster children), was successful in the business world, and has worked toward various social causes in the community. Linda has been a lifelong student of metaphysics, including the spiritual traditions of Judaism, Buddhism, Christianity, Hinduism, and Sufism. She was recently recognized as teacher of dharma by Sensei Ogui and given the dharma name *Shaku Muge Kou* (Follower of Buddha Unhindered Light).

Linda has worked with many masters, on the material plane as well as the higher planes. Her gift of channeling higher levels of consciousness has born fruit in three books that we have written in collaboration with the Ascended Master St. Germain.[1] Linda is currently working on a book with an autobiographical focus.

Our work: Over the past seven years Linda and I have been developing a unique body of knowledge and skills that we named *Psychoenergetic Healing*. We now have arrived at a point of "maturity" in our work, where we feel ready to share our insights and experiences with others. This book has been

---

[1] The books are entitled *Balancing the Light Within*, *Affirmations and Thought Forms*, and *Angels and Other Beings of Light*. Details about these publications can be found in the Appendix.

written to introduce laypersons, energetic healers, and traditional therapists who have open minds to the exciting territory that lies "beyond psychotherapy."

Contact: You may contact us at the following address: *Institute of Psychoenergetic Healing,* P.O. Box 516, Chagrin Falls, OH 44022. Our e-mail address is *expansion@u-r-light.com;* our web site is *www.u-r-light.com.*

Psychoenergetic Healing: A Brief Introduction

Searching for Better Ways: Can you imagine the practice of medicine before the invention of X-ray machines or microscopes? Would you want to refer someone to a doctor who refuses to consider anything that is not visible to the naked eye? The field of psychotherapy, as it is taught in graduate school today, can be likened to the practice of medicine based on a 19th-century view of the world. While there are many fine, traditionally trained psychotherapists out there, psychotherapy is still very much a "hit or miss" endeavor.

We propose that the practice of psychotherapy (and healing in general) cannot advance significantly without a shift in paradigm, i.e., a fundamental reorientation. Within the established paradigm there is no convincing explanation for phenomena such as the placebo effect, "spontaneous" remissions, psychosomatic illnesses, "miracle cures," healing through prayer or touch, etc. As long as the premises of the healing arts are based on a material or mental -- rather than energetic -- understanding of reality, their efforts resemble attempts to assemble a million-piece puzzle without an idea of the larger picture. In the final analysis, scientific "progress" based on a misunderstanding is like getting better at "barking up the wrong tree."

Psychoenergetic Healing is based on a "new" paradigm that is compatible with ancient wisdom teachings as well as modern sciences. Leading-edge physicists have now come to insights similar to those of ancient mystics: All there is, all matter and all of Creation, is "patterned" energy, vibrating to specific frequencies that distinguish one manifestation of energy from another.

What is Psychoenergetic Healing? All psychological manifestations, such as thoughts, feelings, and behavior patterns, are also "patterned" energy. Effective psychological healing, regardless of the method or technique, occurs when there is a change in the basic energies that charge our feelings, thoughts, memories and habits. While all psychotherapeutic methods are intended to produce such healing, most do not target the energetic level directly.

Psychoenergetic Healing takes into account the fact that human beings are not only physical, emotional, and mental beings, but also, and most essentially, spiritual beings. This truth is not a mere statement of faith; it can be experienced in a direct, tangible manner. No matter what names or interpretations we prefer, a spiritual, healing energy, or Light[2], can be accessed by all human beings regardless of our belief systems and can be utilized effectively for healing on all levels.

---

[2] Throughout the book we have chosen to capitalize the word "Light" when we speak of the Light in general terms; when we speak about a specific light, e.g., a blue light, we chose not to capitalize the word.

The practitioner of Psychoenergetic Healing uses a variety of techniques that affect the mental and emotional energies on a fundamental level, thus going directly to the source of the individual's discomfort. While going to the core of the matter may be a frightening thought to many, it is actually a very healing, safe, efficient, and effective method that does *not* require the unbuffered reliving of traumatic memories or painful feelings.

What Happens in a Typical Session? What happens in a session is very much guided by the individual's issues and needs, making each session a unique experience. Most sessions include elements of traditional "talking therapy," expanded upon with work performed in an altered state of consciousness we call "Inner Space"[3] where the client can experience the richness of his or her multidimensional nature. Facilitated by the therapist, the client achieves a heightened state of consciousness in which he or she may become aware of colors, images, thoughts, memories, feelings, or physical sensations, such as pain, heat, weight, etc. The range of experiences in Inner Space is virtually unlimited and may include an awareness of past lives, other dimensions, the presence of beings of Light, and more.

While each client has a different experience, all are able to perceive the flow of energies within. These inner perceptions then guide the course of the healing work. Using what could be called a "psychological X-ray technique," the client can become aware of the core issue and then observe the process of healing on an energetic level as it is occurring. Al-

[3] A more complete definition and explanation of the term "Inner Space" can be found in Chapter 6.

though getting in touch with painful feelings or experiences may cause some temporary discomfort, an energetic shift and tangible relief can often be felt within minutes. Because the client has control over his or her Inner Space and all therapeutic interventions are guided by the client's inner perceptions, this approach to healing is experienced as empowering and safe.

Who Can Benefit From Psychoenergetic Healing? Our experience has shown that Psychoenergetic Healing can be an effective approach regardless of the presenting problem, as all thoughts, memories, feelings, and habits exist as "patterned" energies and can be treated as such. Psychoenergetic Healing has been successfully applied to a wide variety of issues, including anger, fear, depression, addictions, sexual issues, codependency, low self-esteem, traumatic experiences, psychosomatic illnesses, pain, grieving and loss, etc. Clients of all ages, including children and adolescents, have benefited greatly from Psychoenergetic Healing, regardless of their belief systems or prior experience with energy-based healing.

Most of us are not consciously aware of the subtle energies that fuel our behaviors and states of mind at all times, and yet we all have noticed emotional energies in action, such as when we experience intense anger, fear, or resentment. If we do not release and balance negative emotions properly, but instead "sweep them under the rug," they may linger in our emotional body for an unlimited time, causing further disturbance. They may even manifest in physical disease. To gain or maintain a state of harmony and health, it is essential to attend to emotional disharmonies, resolve inner conflicts, and release traumatic memories.

Many of our clients have already accomplished a significant amount of inner work, be it emotional or spiritual in nature, and desire to further their growth by addressing those issues that previously seemed intractable. Thus, to benefit from Psychoenergetic Healing, a commitment to growth can be more relevant than the nature of the problem or whether it fits into any traditional diagnostic pigeonhole.

PART I

Metaphysical Foundations of Psychoenergetic Healing

Chapter 1

Fundamental Premises

The new, energy-based paradigm we spoke of in the introductory chapter is, in fact, not so new, after all. Many Eastern philosophers, mystics, and scientists have long espoused an understanding of creation as a sea of energies in motion, existing on many different levels of frequency. While leading-edge physicists may embrace a compatible view of reality, the predominant mind-set of our times is still based on an understanding of reality more closely related to the physics of the 19th century rather than the 21st. Although tempted, I will not launch into a dissertation on this complex subject. You may wish to refer to writers such as David Bohm, Michael Talbot, Fred Alan Wolf and Deepak Chopra[4] who have built a convincing case tracing the lines of thought -- and demonstrating the convergence -- of ancient Eastern and modern Western views of reality.

[4] For details, see our reading suggestions in the Appendix.

Review of Basic Premises

To lay a foundation of understanding for our purposes, a condensed review of some of the basic premises of metaphysical teachings is in order. If you are a novice in the study of metaphysics, you would be well advised to go over this section more than once, and to give yourself time to think through its implications.

Let us begin with a simple definition: What is metaphysics? The American Heritage Dictionary has the following to offer: "The branch of philosophy that systematically investigates the nature of first principles and problems of ultimate reality. Metaphysics includes the study of being (ontology) and, often, the study of the structure of the universe (cosmology)."

For our purposes, we would add that we are not interested in metaphysics as a mental exercise motivated by a desire to fill books or gain tenure. We call our work "applied metaphysics": We strive to truly understand, apply and live the principles we espouse. The ultimate test of a philosophy is not its logical consistency and irrefutability, but a very simple question: Does it work?

As we have been shown, there are a limited number of Universal Laws that are rather simple. (This is not to say that they are readily understood by the human mind). Here are some of the truths as we understand and have experienced them:

(1) **There is order in the Universe**. The infinite number of forms and appearances are but variations of an underlying theme. There is uniformity in diversity.

(2) **All of creation is vibration** or "patterned" energy that can be perceived and described as light, sound, or a sensation of vibration.

(3) **There is an infinite number of "frequencies"** that comprise the totality of creation.

(4) **The material world is just one level of reality.** Just as the visible colors or audible tones are only segments of the full spectrum of light or sound, so is the material world only a segment of the totality of creation.

(5) **All of creation originates on the subtle planes.** Material creation is a manifestation of subtle vibrations originating on the higher planes and then transformed into denser material vibrations. A good metaphor for this manifestation process is the transformation of H_2O from humidity to vapor to water to ice, a con*densation* or "crystallization" process.

(6) **"As above, so below"** -- as in heaven, so on earth. Macrocosm and microcosm are analogous to one another in their essential constitution, evolution and mode of operation. Again, there is uniformity in diversity.

(7) **Time and space are not what they seem to be.** Our perception of time and space is bound to the human level of awareness. Once we transcend this level of awareness, the limits of time and space that appear so real to the human mind dissolve. (This is a vast and complicated topic, which we will set aside for the time being.)

(8) **All is connected to everything,** and all is affected by everything. There is oneness, despite the illusion of separation.

(9) **All of creation stems from Infinite Source, and all that exists remains a part of it.** The concepts of "good" vs. "evil," "God" vs. "the devil" are based on the illusion of separation.

(10) **Change is the order of the Universe.** We are constantly changing and evolving, and that is true both for the macrocosm and the microcosm.

For those of you who are not used to thinking in abstract metaphysical terms, please be patient with yourselves. You may wish to go over this condensed version of "Metaphysics 101" a few more times before you have a better understanding of its implications. We also recommend titles for further reading in the back of this book.

We Are Living in a Time of Radical Change

We are, indeed, living in interesting times. A tide of change is washing over every fiber of our being, touching every strand of the fabric of life as we know it. This change we are participating in goes to the root of our thinking, feeling, and mode of operation; thus, it is truly *radical* [5] in its nature and scope.

Many attempts have been made to explain the underlying dynamics of this time of transition from a metaphysical perspective. Once again, we will try to give a condensed and necessarily simplified outline of our understanding.

---

[5] "Radical" is derived from the Latin word for root, *radix*.

(1) While the Creator is beyond duality, **Creation exists only within duality**. This duality can be thought of as yin and yang, male and female, negative and positive, light and darkness, etc. Another way of understanding the essence of Creation is to conceive of it as the friction between two forces, the forces of expansion and contraction. In the emotional domain, the force of contraction in its most fundamental expression is experienced as fear, and the force of expansion in its most fundamental expression is experienced as love. In the mental domain, contraction corresponds to judgment, separation, "ego," etc. Expansion corresponds to acceptance, oneness, and surrender of "ego."

(2) **The Universe is changing its balance of expansion and contraction** in a cyclical manner (it is breathing in and out, so to speak). These cycles span long periods of time (according to some belief systems, about 26,000 years). After a long cycle of contraction, we are now at the beginning of a period of expansion.

(3) For a long time, life on planet Earth was dominated by an excess of "masculine" or yang energies. **It is time for a rebalancing and the reemergence of the "feminine"** or yin energies.

(4) Astrologically speaking, **our solar system as a whole is moving from the Piscean age**, which lasted about 2,000 years, **into the age of Aquarius**, which brings with it a major shift in the prevalent energies.[6] While most of us may have heard these terms,

[6] Furthermore, we are currently experiencing the advent of a Pluto-based cycle that occurs every 250 years. This cycle coincides with one that occurs only every 26,000 years: The magnetic north pole is moving toward

none can truly comprehend what this process entails. In what may be called a huge cosmic experiment, planet Earth -- and with it, all of humanity -- is moving into uncharted territory, creating a new reality for all.

Let me try to summarize the changes in a nutshell: The **Piscean age** was characterized by (1) **fear**, e.g., fear of lack or loss of love, power or material possessions; (2) **manipulation** of relationships, one's own personality, one's circumstances, or the environment; (3) **dominion** over nature, animals, and fellow humans.

The **Aquarian age** is characterized by (1) **trust** based on one's connection to Source; (2) **equality** among all living things; (3) **love** and acceptance of self and others instead of judgment; (4) **freedom** of all to live life as determined by their own nature, i.e., as a full expression of their Totality.

This brief characterization of the different ages cannot do justice to the complexity of the many levels of change that we are currently undergoing. After all, this transition leads us into uncharted territory. But from the little that has been said so far, you can see easily that moving from the old mode of operation into the new is nothing short of radical. And you can also assume that the transition will not always be smooth and easy -- neither for Mother Earth, nor the humans dwelling upon her.

---

direct alignment with Polaris, commonly known as the North Star. In addition, a little known but significant lunar cycle of 40,000 years is currently coming to completion. Although we have insufficient experience with astrological events of this magnitude and intensity, one can safely state that these are no ordinary times. (We thank Kristina Strom for her astrological expertise.)

It is Time for a New Paradigm

Another characteristic of the times we live in is the significant increase in higher-vibrational energies permeating this part of the universe with ever-increasing intensity. In fact, these higher-vibrational energies are the driving force behind the radical changes described above. The influx of higher vibrations accelerates the frequencies prevalent on the earth plane. Consequently, the gap between material and non-material levels of vibration is diminishing. The veil that used to separate the two domains is thinning and becoming increasingly more permeable. Thus, more and more human beings are becoming aware of the multidimensional nature of reality. Concepts such as energy fields, auras, spirit communication, intuitive perception, healing energies, etc., are gradually entering mainstream consciousness.

A new view of reality demands changes on many levels, including the way we approach physical and emotional healing. When medicine discovered the microscopic levels of reality, such as the cell, genes, microbes, and bacteria, the practice of medicine had to change drastically. We are now at a similar juncture in the practice of the healing arts. We can no longer ignore the many dimensions of our being that transcend earth-plane thinking and perception. It is time to recognize that we are more than what, for a long time, we thought we were, specifically in the Western world. *It is time to remember and honor the fact that we are multidimensional beings of Light* having a human experience. Hence, it is time to accommodate our mode of operation as healers to this realization and to the new realities of the Aquarian age.

We are given an opportunity to assist in bringing these new realities into full expression on the earth plane. We do not subscribe to the concept of a "mission" assigned to an individual incarnating on planet Earth. We do believe, however, that we incarnate into a certain time and place based on choices we have made on the level of our Higher Self.[7] If we listen to our heart, we can know what those choices were and how to play our chosen part in the birthing process of a new age.

---

[7] The term "Higher Self" will be explained in the following chapter.

Chapter 2

The Multidimensional Nature of Human Beings

Very few human beings fully understand their true natures while living in a physical body. This is not completely surprising. During a physical existence we are very much caught up in the world of appearance as perceived with our five senses and interpreted by our human mind. It is as if we feel locked into one FM radio station, forgetting that our receiver could also pick up AM, short wave, CB and ham radio frequencies, if only we chose to change the dial.

From a metaphysical perspective, however, who we are in our essence is not limited to what we are perceiving with our senses or thinking in our minds. Let us briefly review some basic assumptions about the nature of human beings.

> (1) We are not limited to what we appear to be. Human beings are more than the sum of their body parts, more than a biological organism made of skin and bones.
>
> (2) The human body can be understood as a condensed cloud of "patterned" energy. The physical body is only one segment of the full spectrum of vibrations that comprise the totality of our being.
>
> (3) In addition to the physical body, human beings are composed of interpenetrating energy fields of lesser density, often identified as emotional, mental, and spiritual bodies.

(4) There is no real separation or delineation between the energy fields that are "ours" and those that are "not ours." All is interconnected. All energy fields have an effect on all others, within our material and subtle bodies as well as beyond.

(5) We are constantly "communicating" and exchanging energies with the energy fields around us and within us through our "subtle anatomy" such as the aura, the chakra system, and the meridians (see below for details). We are, in other words, like radio stations that receive and transmit constantly on many different wavelengths.

When we perceive the true nature of the human being to be a multidimensional energy field without fixed boundaries and in constant communication with surrounding energy fields, we can understand more easily how and why we are inevitably affected by changes in the prevailing frequencies. Likewise, we can also understand how our own energy fields affect all others. As we stated above, "all is connected to everything and all is affected by everything."

More About the Human Energy Field

Although the human energy field is not visible to the physical eye, it can be perceived by all of us, to one degree or another, when we open ourselves to our inner vision. Here are some of the basic facts about the human energy field.

Chakras

Human beings can be likened to radio stations that are constantly broadcasting and receiving information. There are specialized centers in the human body that function not unlike satellite dishes, each specializing in a certain frequency. These centers are most commonly called by the Sanskrit word "chakra," which means "wheel of light." In addition to "communicating" with the sea of energies surrounding and penetrating each human form, the chakras play an important role in orchestrating the flow of energies in the physical and the subtle bodies. Generally speaking, the chakras give life force to the organs and glands within their physical and functional proximity. For optimal health on all levels, it is important that all chakras be open and spinning at their respective frequencies in harmony and balance. If the chakras are no longer providing an entrance for life force into the physical body, the physical body ceases to function.

Auras and Subtle Bodies

In addition to possessing a physical body we are surrounded and penetrated by energy fields customarily called "auras" or "subtle bodies." These fields can be photographed and demonstrated in various ways. Auras are of varying frequency, color, form, and degree of expansion, constantly fluctuating in some regards while stable in others. To use a spatial metaphor, one could think of the aura as a set of Russian stacked dolls. This metaphor is to some degree misleading, however, as each layer interpenetrates all others, just as radio waves coexist in the same space.

According to the various teachings and traditions, the subtle bodies can be classified by frequency (for instance, etheric double, lower and higher astral bodies, etc.) or by function. We have found it helpful to distinguish functionally between our physical, emotional, mental, and spiritual bodies. For optimal health on all levels, these bodies need to be fully developed and in alignment and balance with one another.

The Meridian System

The basis of all Eastern traditions of healing is some concept of life force. This energy is called "prana" in the Indian tradition, and "chi," "qi," or "ki" in the Japanese and Chinese traditions. The latter is best known in the West for its system of energy channels (called meridians) that are the "anatomical" basis for the practices of acupuncture and acupressure. Most, but not all, of the more than 1,000 acupuncture points are located on one of the 14 meridians that form a complex network of energy lines throughout the body. Direct manipulation of the flow of energy through insertion of needles, pressure, or the burning of herbs (moxibustion) has long been the focus of traditional Chinese medicine. More recently, the meridian system has come to prominence in various Western healing arts, such as Applied Kinesiology (AK), Neuro-Emotional Technique (N.E.T), Touch for Health, and the like. Over the past decade or two, in the field of psychotherapy, we have seen the emergence of many treatment methods that are based on the meridian system, including Thought Field Therapy (TFT), Emotional Freedom Techniques (EFT), or the Tapas Acupressure Technique (TAT).[8]

[8] We will discuss these techniques in greater detail in Chapter 22.

Other Maps of the Human Energy Anatomy

In addition to the terms and concepts introduced in the paragraphs above, there are numerous other systems and traditions that deserve to be acknowledged. To name a few, there are the energy lines posited in Reflexology or reflex zone therapy and the complex systems underlying the practices of Polarity therapy or Jin Shin Jyutsu. In fact, each healing tradition seems to have developed a somewhat unique map of the territory. To draw a parallel, an orthopedic surgeon is likely to focus on different aspects of the anatomy than would, for instance, an internist, endocrinologist, or neurologist. This is not to imply, however, that the anatomical charts of a neurologist are incompatible with those of an orthopedic surgeon. They are simply different aspects of the whole.

For the practitioner of Psychoenergetic Healing, the chakra system appears to be the most relevant part of the human energy anatomy. Thus, we will discuss the major chakras in greater detail in a later chapter. In addition, the meridian system, which forms the basis of various tapping and acupressure techniques, is also very useful. Since all is energy, we should not rigidly adhere to one system at the exclusion of another; all the various maps may be useful in navigating the many layers of the human energy field.

Our Totality: Beyond the Human Energy Field

We have said that a human being is more than an organism of flesh and bones, and we have discussed some basic ideas about the human energy field. But there is more: There are major portions of what we are in our totality that go beyond the human energy field. In fact, the human portion of our being is just a minuscule fraction of our totality. It is no more than a single cell[9] in a huge organism. These aspects of our totality have been addressed by many names, such as our "Divine Essence," our "God-Self," or our "Higher Self." As beings of light, human beings exist on many planes or levels of vibration simultaneously, with only the lowest frequencies bound to time and space. Our totality comprises light in its lowest vibration (the physical body), light in its highest vibration (our oneness with the Infinite Source), and many frequencies in between. For the sake of simplicity and convenience, let us call those aspects of our totality that transcend time and space and exist on higher-vibrational levels our Higher Self. The Higher Self contains the essence of our existence since the beginning of time; it is the mastermind behind all of our experiences; and it is the direct connection to Infinite Source.

All aspects of our totality are in constant communication. This interchange, of course, is strongly influenced by the receptivity and permeability of our subtle bodies. The greater the balance throughout our human energy field, the easier it is to be in harmony throughout all our totality.

---

[9] This metaphor does not imply that the human portion is insignificant. As the recent advances in cloning have illustrated, a single cell contains all the information needed to form a complete organism.

Chapter 3

The Grand Scheme, Reincarnation, and Karma

The Grand Scheme

In the previous chapter we touched on some fundamental questions: What is the nature of the era we are living in? What is the nature of human beings? In our quest to sketch the larger picture we shall not shy away from the question of the purpose of the human experience. Of course, there are many attempts to give an answer, some more definitive than others. Our own version of the "grand scheme" could be outlined as follows:

First, we acknowledge that we cannot fully comprehend with our human mind the purpose of life in general or our experience of it. Our mind is simply not capable of comprehending a reality that goes far beyond the limits of the mind. If we wish to grasp even the shadow of an answer we need access to our Higher Self. Through our Higher Self an answer may be "known," even if our mind cannot grasp or communicate it. Thus, we can only talk about the grand scheme in approximate terms.

Our totality spans the widest possible range of frequencies, from oneness with Infinite Source to the greatest sense of separation from Infinite Source that we could imagine. No animal would ever feel as separated from Infinite Source as most human beings do. The hallmark of the human experience as we currently know it is this sense of separation. We have "forgotten" that we are, in truth, connected to One and All and, even more, that we are one with One and All.

Human life could be called a grand experiment in consciousness. While all life is imbued with consciousness, human beings are unique insofar as they have chosen to cultivate a frequency of consciousness that is mired in the illusion of separation. The more we suffer from the consequences of this illusion, the more we are driven to rediscover the oneness we have seemingly lost. *All human experience is designed to afford us an opportunity to find again what has, in truth, never been lost.*

In this mind-boggling experiment in consciousness, we are co-creators who have been given the right to exercise free will. We can venture as far away from Infinite Source as we choose, but we can never be apart from Infinite Source. This setup makes for the most interesting and abundant manifestations of *maya*, or cosmic illusion.

And this may be about as far as our human mind will take us. Why is there life? Why is there consciousness? Why is there *maya*? It just is . . . .

Reincarnation

If the purpose of human experience is to return to an awareness of our oneness with Infinite Source, it would be a cruel joke if we had only one lifetime to reach that goal. No matter how long we may live, most of us don't even come close to such a realization. And how could we experiment with the myriad consequences that result from a consciousness of separation if a mere 50 or 80 years were all we had? Obviously, our version of the grand scheme would make little sense without the concept of reincarnation.

Let us describe our understanding of this concept in simple terms: The eternal portion of our totality, which we called Higher Self, delegates an offspring of itself to go to school on the material plane in a human body. In the classroom called "life," each being undergoes a learning process according to an individualized curriculum. The principal in this school is the being's Higher Self, which supervises the curriculum in collaboration with higher-vibrational beings (the superintendents, so to speak) and in accordance with the laws set forth by Infinite Source (the legislature). The principal respects the free will of the student but insists on the supreme goal of learning and growing. If a student refuses to learn a lesson, the same lesson will be presented to him or her again and again in various versions and guises -- until the student is tired of avoiding growth, and decides to tackle the lesson.

Most of us are inclined to avoid growth and change, even if our resistance comes at a high price. Only when the pain becomes intolerable are we willing to do our homework and learn our lessons. The prevalence of learning through painful experiences, of course, is not due to some cruel divine law; it is simply the consequence of our habits and our "forgetfulness." Our Higher Self is primarily interested in our progress as student in the school of life, and not so much in our comfort. Like a wise and benevolent parent, the Higher Self orchestrates experiences for the student that provide the greatest growth opportunities for the highest good of all -- even if the student fights it tooth and nail.

Obviously, no student enters the school of life as a blank page; we all bring some characteristics, dispositions, and attributes with us as we enter this plane. (Parents who have more than one child may not need to be convinced of this assumption.) Not only do we bring innate characteristics to a new embodiment, we also subscribe to a comprehensive curriculum for that particular lifetime. Both are intricately intertwined and in no way accidental.[10]

What we are is determined by what we were and what we shall become. Using the school metaphor again, whether we go on to learn 11th grade math is determined by our performance in 10th grade math and our aspirations for our educational future. Eventually, all students have to master all subjects, but each one completes the curriculum in a unique order and at a unique pace.

It requires numerous incarnations through eons of time until we have learned enough to graduate from the school of life on earth. To be precise, we don't really learn anything new, we only learn to remember what we already know. Our graduation from a life in a human body, however, is not the end of the "grand experiment in consciousness." In fact, there is no end to the expansion of consciousness -- just as there is no end to the expansion of the physical universe.

Karma

While each student has been given free will, the school of life only seems to be anarchic. We learn our lessons within the parameters of the Law of Karma, also known as the Law of

---

[10] Obviously, we do not believe in the idea of a genetic lottery. Our phenotype and personality traits are not the expression of a random recombination of DNA but of a finely crafted blueprint designed on the higher planes. The concepts of "coincidence" and "randomness" are convenient and widely-accepted excuses for a lack of true understanding.

Cause and Effect or the Law of Balance. Most religious traditions have based their ethical reasoning on some version of this law (for instance, "whatever a man sows, that he will also reap" (Gal 6:7) or the Golden Rule). According to such teachings, it is how we use our free will -- i.e., the intent behind our thoughts and actions -- that is the deciding factor in producing "good" or "bad" effects at some later day in one's life, at the time of judgment, or in another lifetime, depending on the specific religious tradition.

While such reasoning may be legitimate in the context of an effort to give ethical guidance, it may also be somewhat misguided. A slightly more neutral, less value-laden interpretation of the Law of Karma sees it only as the Law of Balance, providing us opportunities to "experience the other side," accepting all experiences and rejecting none. This viewpoint would deny that there are "good" or "bad" experiences, and affirm that there are only opportunities to learn.

Which interpretation is right? While *all* experiences are part of the grand experiment in consciousness, and thus *all* are principally neutral and valid, from a human point of view some causes and effects are clearly more pleasant than others. We should not forget, however, that the goal is learning, not comfort. And as students of life, we know that our most painful experiences often prove to be our best teachers.

One could also think of karma as referring to debits and credits on our cosmic bank account. This perspective includes "good" karma as well as "bad," the latter being the kind of karma that most would be concerned with in this context. We design each incarnation based on a balance sheet that lists imbalances with certain other individuals that we intend to address during a specific lifetime. This purpose is one of the factors entering into the design of a lifetime's curriculum. Another factor would be the spiritual and karmic agreements with other souls that our Higher Self negotiated on the higher planes prior to our incarnation. These may be agreements to help a fellow soul advance on his or her spiritual path or to provide opportunities for learning and balancing of karma for others.

Just as a businessman does not expect debits and credits to balance at the end of each day, but rather is striving for a balance over a longer period of time, so human beings do not reach a karmic balance within one lifetime. Instead, the karmic balance is being achieved over many incarnations. If we observe seeming injustices -- some "get away with murder" while others experience inexplicable suffering -- we should remind ourselves that ultimately, all is in perfect order. Lest this more "objective" view sounds callous, we should keep in mind, of course, that wisdom and compassion in the face of suffering -- seeing yourself as one with all others -- are of utmost importance.

Furthermore, we should try to look beyond the human preference for comfort that underlies our judgment of events as "good" or "bad." Just as eating ice cream and pastries every day is more pleasant than healthy, having a lifetime of ease and comfort may not truly be for our highest good. It is wiser to relinquish all judgment of what is "good" or "bad" for us or others, as we can never truly know a person's karmic agenda or what is for that person's highest good.

We would misunderstand the Law of Karma if we equated it with some version of the Old Testament's rule: ". . . as he has done it shall be done to him, fracture for fracture, eye for eye, tooth for tooth" (Lev 24:20). Correctly understood, there is no element of vengeance or punishment in the Law of Karma. Karmic law does not "condemn us" to live down the consequences of our actions. Indeed, the karma we decide to live out in a certain lifetime is based on choices we make on the level of our Higher Self, which decides what lessons we need to learn for our own soul growth and greater understanding.

Our human mind cannot fully comprehend the karmic choices that we make on the higher planes. We simply need to trust that all is designed to advance us on our paths. We can, however, work toward transcending our karma by actively pursuing the lesson we have set out to learn. Once we learn the lesson, once we heal the issue we have had, within ourselves and/or with another person, there is no need to perpetuate a particular karmic drama. When a student has learned the material, he or she can move on.

Balancing of karma with another person may occur solely on the higher planes. Restitution or balancing on the material plane is not necessary. As the veils between the higher and lower planes are lifting, access to the higher planes can be achieved ever more easily. This now allows us to heal and release much of our karma in other ways than the path of suffering that seemed so inevitable in the past. We are, indeed, at the threshold of a new time that allows us to close the books of the past. More easily than ever before, we now have the opportunity to choose to leave our karma behind and begin a new book altogether, rather than add yet another chapter to the old story.

Chapter 4

Co-creation and Manifestation

Many have heard the formula that "you create your own reality." While this has become a mantra-like staple of New Age thought, it is an idea not well understood. When we find ourselves in a painful situation, we may doubt that we really *chose* to experience such pain. No matter what we proclaim, when we become really miserable and uncomfortable, we tend to see ourselves as victims of adverse circumstances or actions, feeling that others have wronged us, by life, or by God. After all, who would have chosen to go through such an experience?

And yet, there are *no* victims, we *do* have free will, and we *are* the creators or our own reality. The choices, however, aren't necessarily conscious choices of our human mind. These choices may have been made in other lifetimes or before we entered this incarnation. Or they may have been made by our Higher Self in the interest of balancing karma or progressing in the school of life. Remember, comfort is not an important concept for our Higher Self -- but soul growth and expansion is.

It is the Higher Self that chooses a set of parents, relatives, and the time, place and circumstances into which we incarnate. Although some may argue that such a setup places limitations on our choices, there is still ample room for choice all along the way. In fact, in every moment we determine the level of frequency of our thoughts and feelings, and there are myriad opportunities to choose actions, thoughts, feelings, and intentions. And each choice has consequences, whether they are limited to the subtle planes or manifest on the material plane. Rather than thinking in terms of "predetermination," it would be more fitting to speak of a "context" in which the human mind operates and chooses at each moment -- in concert and continuous communication with our Higher Self and the human minds and Higher Selves of others.

So far we have only spoken of choices, as if we had been placed in a giant supermarket with the task of choosing our menu, to the best of our abilities. But this is still a limited concept. To stay in the picture, consider that we are actually co-creating the supermarket itself! Let me try to explain this idea in a metaphor: The world around each individual is like a hologram, or a movie, projected from the center (the individual) onto a spherical screen around that individual. It is part of the grand scheme that we tend to have little awareness of our role as projectionist in the center of our own personal movie theater. Instead, we perceive things as going on "out there" on the screen like a child who gets caught up in a dramatic movie. In reality, the movie originates in the projectionist's booth -- not on the screen where we see it happening.

In a previous chapter, we stated that all of creation is vibration, or Light, and that we are indeed beings of Light. Keeping this fundamental premise in mind, let us continue with the "movie theater projectionist" metaphor: Instead of using light from a light bulb, we use the Light coming from Infinite Source through our Higher Self. Instead of mirrors, prisms, and a strip of celluloid, we use the human energy field, especially the chakras, which can be likened to lenses overlaid with a stack of transparencies, or movie frames. Each chakra contains information imprinted upon it through present and past choices and experiences. We filter the Light coming from our Higher Self through the human energy field and project it onto the screen around us, thus creating our own personal movie experience.

To illustrate this process, let us briefly describe the past life experiences of a 15-year-old male client. This young man had an extensive history of injuries to the head through accidents, dog bites, etc. Initially, he was reluctant to explore what may have been the underlying energetic pattern that resulted in repeated injuries to the same body part. With a little bit of encouragement while working in Inner Space, he was ultimately willing to look into the matter and soon entered a time stream of a recent past life[11]. In that lifetime he was a soldier who was killed on the battlefield by shrapnel that had struck his head. He was able to receive very clear images and to go back to the time preceding his lethal injury. I asked him to perceive his energetic body in that lifetime, and he noticed that the head region showed significant energetic disturbances even before he sustained the head injury (stemming from experiences we do not need to explain at this point). He then stated that it seemed as if the shrapnel had been *magnetically attracted* by the negativity in his head region. Thus, what looked like an "accident" from the outside was actually a manifestation of an energetic disturbance from within.

The observation of this 15-year-old client is by far not singular. In fact, many of our clients are able to perceive repetitive patterns of energetic disturbances through several lifetimes, often resulting in injury or death in past lives and repeated injuries of the same body region in the present life. This observation illustrates that we are indeed the creators of our experiences, and that manifestation originates first on the

---

[11] We will discuss the topic of past life trauma in Chapter 17.

subtle planes -- which is, of course, one of the most central metaphysical tenets.

Chapter 5

Toward a New Paradigm of Healing

This book is about "healing," and it is time to examine and define what this means from a metaphysical perspective (the clinical and technical details will be discussed in the main body of this book). *Healing simply means to shift the balance of energies within an energy field (human or otherwise) toward harmony and higher vibrations, or, conversely, to reduce the prevalence of disharmony and lower vibrations.* As there are no "empty spaces" in an energy field, one shift goes hand in hand with the other.

Having given this fundamental definition, we can move on to some basic points about healing:

(1) All illness and dis-ease, be it mental, emotional or physical, is an expression of an energetic imbalance or disharmony. As all manifestation "steps down" from the subtle to the denser levels of vibration, the presence of a disease indicates an imbalance on the subtle levels.

(2) Healing is a manifestation of increased balance and harmony; as with all manifestations, it, too, originates on the subtle planes. There is no essential difference between physical, emotional, mental, or spiritual healing.

(3) Higher levels of vibration are more harmonious and thus more healing than lower levels. Higher vibrations can be experienced as love, joy, peace, happiness, forgiveness, gratitude, bliss, etc. Lower vibra-

tions are associated with the experience of anger, depression, fear, guilt, shame, greed, etc. The highest levels of vibration are customarily called the spiritual levels.

(4) Effective healing occurs when a more harmonious energy field interacts with a less harmonious frequency, resulting in a transmutation from lower to higher frequency.

(5) An effective healer is someone who channels or emits more harmonious energies and facilitates the transmutation process. Likewise, an effective healing agent is something that emanates more harmonious energies (such as an undisturbed natural environment), something we charge with thoughts of healing (such as a medication or a placebo), or something that contributes to a greater degree of balance (on the physical, emotional, mental, or spiritual level). Effective treatment aims to transform the barriers that were put in place between lower-vibrational energies (for instance, fears) and higher-vibrational energies such as trust or peace, so that the latter can transform the former.

(6) Not all treatment is healing, and not all healing results from treatment. All we need to do to achieve healing is to allow the perfection that already exists on the highest levels of our being to "percolate" down to the level that holds the imbalance. Ultimately, all healing is self-healing.

(7) All healing is possible. If we think of the physical, emotional and mental bodies as clouds of "patterned" energies, there is virtually no limit to the creation of harmony. In other words, nothing is "writ-

ten in stone," as all is in flux and constantly changing, similar to clouds in the sky.

(8) Healing may take many forms; it is unique for each individual and situation. The healing process occurs on many levels simultaneously. Although we often have preconceived ideas about the desirable outcome, our human minds are not equipped to accurately judge the outcome of a healing process as "success" or "failure."

(9) Healing is an ongoing process. Just as our physical cells are continuously breaking down and continuously being repaired, so is energetic healing a never-ending process. The notion that you are either healthy (i.e., health defined as the absence of any diagnosable disease), or sick (defined as the presence of a diagnosable disease) is simplistic and mistaken. Emotional, physical, or energetic health is a matter of degree, not an either-or dichotomy.

(10) Given humanity's level of evolution at this point in history, all of us carry a certain degree of imbalance and disharmony, reflected in a disturbance of the flow of subtle energies throughout the human energy field. Thus, all of us are in need of healing, on one level or another.

As we stated earlier, our corner of the universe and all that is within it are moving toward a higher level of vibration, which makes higher-vibrational frequencies ever more readily accessible. Future advances in the healing arts will be achieved most effectively by using those energies in a systematic manner that hold the greatest healing power, such as love, joy, peace, forgiveness, gratitude, bliss, and other spiritual frequencies.

We predict that during this period of transition, we will be observing more and more illnesses and dis-eases that will not respond well to treatment limited to gross material frequencies, such as the prescription of pharmaceuticals. As the health care establishment will find itself increasingly overwhelmed and impotent, practitioners who use higher-vibrational approaches to healing will be increasingly in demand.

PART II

The Practice of Psychoenergetic Healing

Chapter 6

The Nature of Inner Space

In the initial paragraphs introducing Psychoenergetic Healing we used the term "Inner Space." What do we mean by this?

(1) Inner Space denotes a heightened state of awareness, in which the client taps into his or her intuitive knowing and opens to a way of perceiving that could be called "extrasensory," in the sense that it does not rely on the perception of outer stimuli. Instead, the client opens to an *inner* seeing, hearing, sensing, or knowing.

(2) Inner Space also refers summarily to the levels of reality that can only be perceived in such a heightened state of awareness. Thus, the term denotes a way of perceiving a reality, as well as the reality itself.

While this may sound like a "blurred" definition, it is with intent. We do not subscribe to the concept of an "objective" reality separate from the "subjective" observer. Such a pre-Einsteinian notion is still a popular (mis-) understanding of the scientific paradigm. Instead, for our purposes we assume that there is no reality outside the observer who perceives it.

Inner Space is as vast and unlimited as outer space. Therefore, it is not easy to define Inner Space, at least not in affirmative terms. It is easier to state what Inner Space is *not*: It is not limited by the notion of time and space and the usual modes of perception operative in every-day consciousness. This fact has significant implications.

Let us talk about *space* first. In Inner Space, our awareness can focus on *any* place *within* our body. For instance, we may "see" into a nerve or perceive the flow of energy within our toes. We may also focus on *any* place *around* our body, such as our aura, our home, the whole planet, or anywhere in outer space. And we may choose to perceive the flow of energies in any distant place or person, allowing for long-distance perception and healing.

To go even further, we may perceive an object in Inner Space that has no relation to any objective space at all. A typical example would be someone who perceives stairwells or doorways within one's heart. Obviously, no person *really* has such objects in his or her heart -- but they are not uncommonly found in Inner Space. Such purely "virtual" perceptions may frequently be observed in Inner Space. They should not be dismissed as annoying hallucinations or "random noise." For the trained observer, they are useful pieces of information and "grist for the mill" in the healing process.

In regard to *time*, Inner Space is just as interesting. Understanding the true nature of time is not easy for a human mind that is accustomed to thinking in linear terms, with the past preceding the present, which is preceding the future. As we achieve access to the higher planes of reality in Inner Space, time does not have the characteristic of a one-way street. In fact, rather than thinking of "time as a vector," a more apt metaphor may be "time as a sphere."

Imagine that all that has ever happened, all that is happening, and all that will ever happen is "located" on the surface of a sphere of glass. Then, picture yourself sitting at the center of the sphere and perceiving any event you like by training your eyes on any given point "in time." Since all points on the surface of a sphere are equidistant from its center, all points can be observed equally easily, regardless of their relation to the past-present-future illusion that our minds invented to organize our reality.

What does this mean for the purpose of healing? While in Inner Space, the client can easily perceive events that happened many years ago, appeared forgotten, or were outside the conscious awareness, such as preverbal or perinatal experiences. Furthermore, events that happened *in utero*, at conception, or before conception on the higher planes may also be perceived. And then there is the wide field of past lives and their effect on the present lifetime. As weird as it may sound, when working in Inner Space it is quite possible to heal traumatic events from the past, including past lives. There *is* truth in the bumper sticker slogan, "It is never too late to have a happy childhood!" (More about that in a later chapter.)

Besides dealing with events from the past, clients occasionally choose to use Inner Space for a look into the future. This may be particularly useful in the context of decision-making and weighing of alternatives. Occasionally, clients may have "psychic" visions of the future that answer an inner desire for knowing but are not necessarily related to the healing of a present-time issue. In general, however, the option of looking into the future[12] is relatively rarely chosen.

[12] It should also be noted at this point that when we speak of "looking into the future" we do not imply a fatalistic notion of the future as predeter-

Another characteristic of Inner Space is its unifying frame of reference. One of the basic assumptions underlying Psychoenergetic Healing is the premise that "all of creation is vibration," meaning that patterned energy in motion is all there is. This truth is much more easily perceived in Inner Space. When we deal with a physical problem, such as a broken leg or abdominal cramps, we look at the area of discomfort from within, perceive the flow of energies that are at the core of the discomfort, and then we use healing energies for physical symptoms in quite the same manner as we would in the healing of mental, emotional, or spiritual issues.

For the skeptic, let us share this little anecdote: One of my (Martin) clients was a chiropractor whose clinical specialty was pain management. One morning he called to cancel his appointment because of sudden unbearable pain in his shoulder that had kept him from sleeping. That morning he had seen a medical doctor for a cortisone injection, which had brought him no relief. When he called to cancel, I asked him to come anyway. I was quite certain that we could take care of his pain -- which we did in less than ten minutes.

In summary, Psychoenergetic Healing goes beyond the limits of traditional psychotherapy. Its scope of application includes the healing of physical, emotional, mental, and spiritual issues. And it allows healing beyond time and space, including the healing of past life trauma as well as long-distance healing of others.

---

mined. Rather, we see the future as an array of potential realities subject to our choices.

Chapter 7

The Structure of Psychoenergetic Healing Sessions

The First Session: Assessment and Treatment Planning

Obviously, the initial session differs from all subsequent sessions insofar as there is more time devoted to getting to know each other, establishing rapport and trust, explaining the nature of the work, and getting a sense of the client's needs and history. Considerable time may be spent taking a person's health history, as many of our clients have had numerous health challenges, operations, and accidents, or are taking medications. We also tend to ask about any traumatic experiences, losses, or separations, or a family history of substance abuse -- or any other kind of abuse -- as well as past treatment experiences. However, there are no binding rules for the initial session along the lines of a conventional "intake interview" with its emphasis on information gathering, psychological assessment, diagnosis, and treatment planning.

In this line of healing work, the gathering of factual information has a different significance than in traditional psychotherapy for several reasons. First, much of the really important information may not be accessible through a simple interview as we may not be conscious of the true impact of certain experiences from this or past lifetimes. Second, the presenting problem may turn out to be relatively marginal in comparison to other issues the client may discover in the course of the healing journey. For instance, a client came for treatment of his cigarette addiction. Additionally, although an accomplished body builder, he had a respiratory condition that had severely limited his lung capacity. In the course of treatment, we discovered that the impact of two life experiences, a near-drowning at age four and the traumatic loss of a sibling, had created energetic blocks that fueled his addiction and restricted his breathing. Once we had worked through these and a few other issues, some of them stemming from past lives, he was able to free himself from his addiction.[13]

Thus, while conventional treatment planning takes a back seat in Psychoenergetic Healing, the process is, by far, not a random shot into the dark. Our philosophy of a "treatment plan" is based on three assumptions: (1) The client is a multidimensional being of light who potentially can make use of many levels of awareness. (2) The healing process is guided by many factors, known and unknown, and will unfold *in perfect order*. (3) The "treatment team" includes the client's and the healer's Higher Selves as well as all the beings of light[14] connected to either. We are never alone in the process, and we cannot orchestrate it from our position of relative ignorance. Thus, there is a treatment plan in effect, but we may not be privy to it with our human minds.

To highlight the difference between conventional approaches to a first session interview and our work, let me share what I (Martin) have told many first-time clients of mine. After a brief introduction of myself and my office procedures I invite them to tell me *anything they like*. I may tell them that I would be interested in their reasons for coming, as well as

---

[13] We discuss energetic blocks in Chapter 12 and addictions in Chapter 17.

[14] Please refer to our book *Angels and Other Beings of Light* for additional information.

some background information regarding their living situation, children, parents, spouse, work, etc. I may also suggest that they tell me some of their history, including childhood experiences, health issues, or important life events. And then I tell them that they do not need to tell me anything at all, and that we could start with the healing work without preliminaries, as the process would reveal the important information, anyway.

There are at least four reasons why I may ask for information of the kind listed above: (1) It helps the client to introduce him/herself and to establish a relationship. (2) The rules of my profession, as well as those of the insurance industry, require history and diagnosis. (3) Being aware of health problems and life events can give me an initial overview and a mental map relative to the chakra system (see below for details); it may also provide a useful timeline of events. (4) Having some biographical background information can help in piecing the puzzle together when we discover energetic blocks while working in Inner Space. For example, there may be a big black ball of sadness in the third chakra that the client may not be able to understand easily. If I have prior knowledge of, for instance, the parents' divorce at age three, I may suggest that the client think about that event and check how the black ball responds to such thoughts.

In summary, conducting some sort of initial assessment may be quite useful for a number of reasons, but it is not a prerequisite to a healing intervention! The work in Inner Space has its own logic, which overrides any psychological or therapeutic conceptualizations. It is important to remain open and flexible to what "surprises" may be revealed in Inner Space.

Psychoenergetic Healing: More Than a "Talking Cure"

Traditionally, most schools of psychotherapy consider talking central to the task. Thus, the content and style of the therapeutic exchange is often fairly regulated, depending on what is considered curative in any particular school of thought. In Psychoenergetic Healing, the content and style of our conversations may vary widely, ranging from client-centered listening to Socratic dialogue, from sharing of personal experiences to philosophical discourse. More important than a specific plan or method is the therapist's ability to listen simultaneously to both the client and his or her inner guidance -- and then to trust the process as it unfolds. This framework allows a great deal of latitude and flexibility, which helps in keeping the work fresh and innovative.

Sometimes we may just sit and listen, occasionally offering a thought or comment. Other times we use the material presented as a launching pad for a discourse aimed at shedding light on a client's issues from a perspective of "applied metaphysics." For instance, we may discuss issues such as judgment of self and others, empowerment versus a sense of victimization, confusion of the mind versus guidance from the heart, the question of "sin" and karma, and similar topics.[15] In summary, in Psychoenergetic Healing talking is undoubtedly important, but it is just one of many tools in the box.

---

[15] More about the role of teaching and coaching can be found in Chapter 21.

The Basic Structure of a Healing Session

First, it is important to emphasize that there is almost no hard and fast rule about *anything* in a Psychoenergetic Healing session. If circumstances require it or your intuition demands it, be open to flexibility and change in *all* you do. Having said that, let us begin to organize the subject matter at hand by outlining a typical session. The length of a session varies from one hour to -- in rare cases -- three hours.[16] Sessions with children tend to be shorter than adult sessions. Most adult sessions take about two hours. However, shorter sessions may be less taxing for the client, reducing premature dropout due to a sense of being overwhelmed. Typically, about half the time is spent in "talking mode," the other half in Inner Space.

In the first part of the session, the therapist reestablishes contact, asks how the client has been doing, whether there are any changes in the presenting problem, any new observations, awarenesses, insights, challenges, physical symptoms, and so on. What we talk about is largely determined by the moment, taking into consideration the client's needs, interests, beliefs, personality style, and many other factors.

Anywhere between 10 and 90 minutes into the session, we may choose to shift gears and enter into Inner Space. Before we do so, there is often a bathroom break to avoid disruptions later on. After the work in Inner Space, clients are often tired or emotionally exhausted. Other times they may feel elated, peaceful, and expansive. We routinely ask our clients how they feel when they come out of Inner Space. If the client

---

[16] When scheduling clients, we often remind them to eat lightly before the session so that they can sustain the needed concentration. Clients who are hungry and/or tired are harder to work with.

feels light-headed or slightly disoriented, there may be a few minutes spent on centering or grounding. Depending on the circumstances, the therapist may work toward a cognitive integration of the experiences the client just had in Inner Space. This may take the form of relating the current session to previous ones or to pertinent biographical experiences or issues that seem to be related to the larger picture. Some sessions may close with specific instructions for "homework" or after-care.[17]

The Role of the Healer

In Psychoenergetic Healing, the role of the healer can be considered a cross between a therapist, teacher, shaman, surgeon, priest, and fellow traveler on the road to healing and growth. The healer's general attitude should be one of respect, love, compassion, wisdom, service, and acceptance. The healing work is based on respect for the client's path and choices. The healer does not attempt to "fix" something in the client as there is, in truth, nothing that needs "fixing"; the client is already perfect as he or she *is*. It is important to understand that we cannot assist in the process of change before we accept what *is* without judgment.

When it comes to working in Inner Space, the healer operates in the role of a coach or pilot, helping to navigate the challenging territory found in Inner Space. While the client provides the "eyes" and "voice," the healer functions as the "brain." He/she interprets the observations voiced by the client

---

[17] Details will be discussed in Chapter 16.

and directs the journey through Inner Space in accordance with his/her inner guidance, intuition, and experience.

Throughout the session it is the healer's task to "hold the space" (i.e., to stay in a higher-vibrational state of mind) by asking for guidance from the Light and by cultivating a consciousness of being a humble vessel of the Light, asking one's own ego needs to step aside, that the highest good may be served.

Chapter 8

A Sample Session

The following is a transcript of a sample session that we present at this point to provide an example of the work that occurs in Inner Space. This session is relatively brief and straightforward; it illustrates only a portion of the techniques described in later sections of this book.

The client and therapist are familiar with one another from previous Psychoenergetic Healing sessions. Thus, little warm-up or introductory work was necessary in preparation for the work in Inner Space. Before we began, the client, a Reiki[18] master in her eighties, had reported persistent pain in her back between her shoulder blades. This pain had been with her since childhood; it was especially pronounced when she was playing piano or typing on a typewriter, and it had gotten worse in recent days whenever she gave Reiki, which requires a similar position of the arms.

After we set up a higher-vibrational energy field and entered Inner Space, the following interchange -- which took about 45 minutes -- ensued:

Martin: Let's take a look at the place where you are feeling the pain.
Alice: There is a black wire or rope or something like that. It runs vertically. It doesn't seem to be connected to anything.
M: How big is the wire or rope?
A: Not very long; it's more like a straw.

---

[18] Reiki is an energy-based healing technique rooted in an ancient eastern tradition.

M: Can we get into that straw?
A: Yes. It gets very narrow.
M: OK. You can focus your awareness like a laser beam, like the size of a pinhead, and then go into the straw.
A: I'm hitting a wall.
M: OK, look around and see what you find, whether you can find a crack in the wall, or a doorway. . . .
A: The straw is going through the wall.
M: Well, if the straw can go through the wall, we can, too.
A: It looks like I'm coming out the other end; it gets lighter towards the other end.
M: OK, let's Roto-Rooter the straw with violet light. . . . Can the violet show up in the straw?
A: Yes, it is cleaning up the straw.
M: Is the straw gone?
A: Well, it seems there is just a shadow of it left.
M: Hmmm. Let's see whether the straw is connected to something, some place from where it is drawing its energy.
A: No, it doesn't seem to. . . .
M: When I asked that question I felt something in my heart. . . . OK, let's go back to where we felt the pain and where there is still a shadow of the straw. . . . When you focus on that spot, what is the first number that comes to mind when I ask this question: How old is the straw?
A: Three. . . . Now I feel something in my heart.
M: What do you notice?
A: It's at the bottom of my heart. It's like a gray mud, like I'm standing in some mud up to my ankles.
M: OK, let's get into that mud. Sink into it as deeply as you can.
A: I'm in it to the knees.
M: Go deeper.

A: I'm sinking into it, I can't breathe! I don't want to go there -- it's scary -- I want to get out of there!
M: You know, that is exactly why we need to go there, go where it is least comfortable. . . . OK, let's go to age three. Think of any situation or time and place that comes to mind around age three. . . . Are you indoors or outdoors? Is it day or night?
A: Nothing really comes to mind. The only thing is a scene that doesn't seem that important. . . .
M: Let's not edit what it is. Just tell me what comes to mind.
A: Well, my father had just come back from the war. We were having breakfast. My parents and my grandparents were sitting in the dining room. I had to eat in the kitchen with the servants. I came into the dining room and crawled under the table. Then I came up between my grandfather's knees and he gave me some of his egg. And my father said, "DON'T DO THAT -- YOU WILL SPOIL HER! -- GO BACK TO THE KITCHEN!" And I didn't understand.
M: So he made this harsh statement, in a harsh voice. A man who really was a stranger to you at that time. . . . Just feel what you felt then, when you heard that.
A: (Starts breathing heavily, sobs silently; I hand her a tissue.) I never thought that really meant anything. . . .
M: Can we bring the violet light into the dining room, fill the whole scene with violet light. . . ? Let all the players be bathed in violet, Grandpa, father, little Alice. . . . Can the violet fill the scene?
A: Yes.
M: And when you feel the violet has done its job, ask for the golden-white light to fill everyone and everything, too. . . . Is the little girl happy again?
A: Yes, she is smiling.

M: OK, let's take the violet Roto-Rooter and work our way into the straw through the connecting pipeline that feeds the straw.
A: OK. . . . It's there. . . . There is no straw anymore. (Takes a few deep breaths.) I feel the energy go to my lower back -- but maybe that's because I have my hands over my belly. . . . (Alice is a Reiki master who frequently channels healing energy through her hands).
M: Let's go there anyway. What do you notice down there?
A: There is a slight pulsing.
M: Go to the spot from where the pulsing seems to be coming.
A: It's a yucky, mustardy yellow there (points to second chakra); it's in concentric circles, with the center being a little darker.
M: Go to the center of the concentric circles where it is darkest and densest. . . . Let's ask again, how old is that spot? What is the first number that comes to mind?
A: Six. I guess I am in first grade.
M: What happened then, when you were in first grade, around age six?
A: A girl from our class was killed in a horrible car accident during lunch break. -- And I was unhappy, alone. There were the other kids [siblings] then, and my parents didn't have time for me. I just felt awful.
M: Was it more this one moment in time when the girl was killed, or was it more the general misery that you felt then?
A: Well, both. The girl was just once, but the other stuff went on for a long time.
M: Let's go to the time when the girl died. What happened then?

A: We had gone home for lunch, and when we got back to school after lunch the teacher broke out in tears and she told us. I didn't know what to do. . . .
M: Did you see the accident?
A: No, I just heard about it in class.
M: And you might have wondered how God would allow all that? (Alice comes from a very religious, fundamentalist family.)
A: I don't know whether I thought about any of that at that time. . . .
M: Well, they [parents] may have talked about the girl now being in Heaven and stuff like that.
A: They probably would have hoped that she'd be "saved. . . ."
M: Now, when you were so unhappy and lonely, no one paying attention to you. . . . Did you think, maybe it would be better if I went to Heaven, too, like the little girl?
A: I'm not sure. I may have, but I don't remember. . . .
M: Sometimes we have this death wish when we feel miserable, even if it's not conscious. Let's just ask for the violet light and maybe the golden light to go through the body and cleanse and heal any thought along those lines that you may have had.
A: Yes, and let us also ask for healing of all the later times when I really had this death wish. . . .
M: OK, let's ask the violet and golden-white lights to sweep through your body and transform any and all of those thought forms, going back through the centuries, as these are ancient patterns that we tend to carry within. . . .
A: All right. . . .
M: OK, take a few really deep breaths and fill yourself with light. See whether there is any block left, either around the belly button or between the shoulders.

A: (Takes a few, very deep breaths.) No, there doesn't seem to be any.
M: How is the belly button?
A: A bright yellow.
M: Happy and shiny?
A: Yes.
M: And the spot between the shoulders?
A: That's fine. I don't sense anything there anymore. (Keeps breathing deeply and slowly.)
M: OK, then. What would be the right healing, sealing color, or set of colors, to seal in our work today?
A: Let's take the golden-white.
M: All right, take it into your whole body, into every cell, molecule, and atom; let it fill all the time and space that we've touched on today.
A: I feel like my whole body is tingling with this golden light.
M: Well, it is. Take your time and take it all in. . . .

Three days after this session, Alice reported that she was feeling an uncommon sense of freedom because she was able to take really deep breaths as hardly ever before. She stated that there was no pain between the shoulder blades anymore and that she was debating whether she should keep an appointment with a chiropractor that she had set up because of her persistent pain. -- Many months later, the pain that Alice had felt for more than 70 years has not returned.

Chapter 9

Accessing Inner Space

The following description of the various stages, concepts, phenomena, and techniques that comprise the body of Psychoenergetic Healing may at times appear disjointed or overwhelming and you may find integrating the information taxing. We have wrestled long and hard with the question of how best to present this material. To use a metaphor, our task is similar to that of a composer who has to put a symphony on paper one note at a time. Your task is similar to that of a conductor who needs to read the individual notes in order to "recreate" the symphony. Please bear with us; we are sure it is worth the effort.

My office is equipped with a comfortable recliner on a swivel base. This setup allows the client to turn away from me and recline. In that position I[19] can fairly easily hold my hands over the client's head, resting my arms on the top of the chair's back. I habitually put a tissue[20] between my hands and the client's head to absorb oils or moisture (most important on hot summer days). Sometimes my hands rest gently on the head, sometimes they hover over the head, allowing the client to move more freely.

---

[19] "I," "my," and "mine" refer to Martin.

[20] Never start this work without a sufficient supply of facial tissues at hand. Things can get very emotional very quickly, and tears are just part of what happens. In fact, I sometimes say to my clients, in jest, "If you don't cry, you'll get your money back."

Before the client enters Inner Space for the first time, I explain my usual mode of operation and ask the client for permission to touch him or her in the manner described above. I also explain that my "channeling" of energy through my hands during the session is not absolutely necessary; in fact, a Psychoenergetic Healing session can be conducted over the phone with someone thousands of miles away. I further explain that I have found that using my hands in this fashion helps to stabilize the heightened state of awareness[21] required for the energetic work, and that it is generally experienced as soothing or nurturing by the client. So far, I have never had a client who was not agreeable or who rejected my "laying on of hands." Again, how you arrange your setting and whether you choose to support the healing work "hands-on" is entirely up to the individual healer; my wife's clients, for instance, sit facing her on a couch, and she does not use her hands in the described manner.

Some first-time clients may come to you with a great deal of apprehension about their ability to perceive the flow of energies within; others may already have an awareness of such and carry little doubt as to their abilities in this regard. When working with first-time clients, it is important to reassure them that all are able to access Inner Space and that it is the healer's responsibility to help them toward this state of awareness. All they need to do is relax and trust the process.

---

[21] An interesting experiment with brain wave monitoring equipment demonstrated a significant change in a subject's brain wave pattern in the direction of deep relaxation following the positioning of my hands above the head, without actually touching the head (to avoid contamination of the electric currents). Upon withdrawl of my hands, the subject's brain waves reverted to the normal pattern.

While accessing Inner Space is easier for some and more difficult for others, we have yet to encounter a client who was completely unable to enter Inner Space. Those clients who have a harder time shifting to another level of consciousness certainly pose a greater challenge and may at times test the healer's skills and patience. But I assure all my first-timers that *anybody* can do this work in Inner Space, and I mean it.

Setting Up a Higher-Vibrational Force Field

The first step in accessing Inner Space is the establishment of a higher-vibrational force field. To avoid all misunderstanding, Inner Space is not just a "mental" state akin to the "subconscious mind" addressed in hypnosis. We are dealing with higher-vibrational energies, not just with thoughts or imagery. To set the stage it is necessary to invoke these energies, a process we call "setting up a higher-vibrational force field." This can be done quite simply through an invocation, prayer, symbol, silent request, or some other way of focusing and expressing one's intent.[22]

When working with children I tend to set up the force field in a silent manner; I may do the same for first-time adult clients, depending on my assessment of their frame of reference. In most cases, however, I speak a standard "formula." I feel that adhering to a formula has a soothing, reassuring effect on both parties. However, I do not suggest that there is any unique magic in the words I have chosen. I encourage you to

[22] Both, Linda and I have observed that when we shift our awareness, there is frequently a physical shift, as well, in the form of a slight burp.

develop your own style that is comfortable for you and your clients.

This is what I normally say:

"So we ask for the reactivation of the golden pyramids[23] of Light over this space, this building, and the entire region and we ask for the help, presence and blessings of the Archangels[24] Gabriel, Uriel, Michael, and Raphael, asking them each to take a side of these pyramids of Light, energizing them and filling them with healing, cleansing, and balancing Light from Source. And we ask for the help, guidance, and inspiration of the ascended and angelic beings, the Christ Light[25], the Divine Mother energy, our Higher Selves, and all other Light Beings wishing to help."

Then I pause and ask the client to relax, breath into the belly, and open to an awareness of a flow from within. For beginners, I explain that such flow may be perceived as a warmth or tingling, as a weight or pain or other physical sensation, as a thought, feeling or image that comes to mind, as an inner sound, or as an inner color. I further explain that most

---

[23] Pyramids of Light are powerful structures of Light that may be used in a variety of ways. Without going into greater detail at this point, suffice it to say that they function like a "magnifying glass" for higher vibrations. -- Linda usually also asks for a crystalline pyramid of Light with a golden capstone to descend into the healing space.

[24] More information on the Archangels, Ascended Masters, and other beings of Light can be found in our book *Angels and Other Beings of Light.*

[25] I am referring to the Christos, or Christ Light, and the Divine Mother energy, not specifically to Jesus, Mary, or any other personage who embodied these energies. Again, our work is essentially nonreligious and nondenominational.

people have the easiest time seeing colors, such as a violet, blue, green, yellow, pink, gold, white, or any other color that comes to mind. Then I encourage the client to report all perceptions without editing, and I wait a little while for a response.

If the client seems to have a hard time picking up an inner vision or perception, I may choose to place the index and middle finger of my right hand on his/her forehead at the area of the "third eye" (the sixth chakra). Then I ask what color he/she perceives as coming from my fingertips. If the client perceives one of the healing colors (see below for a detailed discussion), I ask the client to allow that color to expand and to spread throughout his/her body. If the client reports a black, gray, red, or brown color, we would proceed according to the steps outlined in Chapter 13.

For first-time clients who appear particularly tense, anxious, or "out of touch," I may choose to "prime the pump" with a guided meditation and visualization exercise. Here is what I might say:

> "See yourself sitting under a waterfall of light, golden and white light that is pouring over your body from a source way above your head, a waterfall of light without weight and without noise. This steady stream of healing light is washing over your body, surrounding it with golden-white light and filling it, if you allow. Imagine a funnel or satellite dish on top of your head, funneling the golden-white rays through the fontanel -- where the babies have the soft spot on top of the head -- into your head, filling your head and your forehead, your eyes, nose, and jaws with golden-white light. . . . Then see this light moving down along the spine to the throat, to the area of the Adam's apple, and

> visualize this light filling your throat and neck with a beautiful, healing radiance. . . . Then see this light flowing down along the spine to the level of your heart, filling the heart with golden-white light, radiating out from the heart into the lungs, the chest, and the entire upper body. . . . Then see the golden-white light flowing down along the spine to the midsection of the body, to a place between the sternum and the navel. This beautiful radiance is filling the diaphragm, the stomach, the liver, and all adjacent organs, the entire midsection of the body. . . . Then see this light moving down along the spine to the level of the navel, filling the belly button, the bladder, the uterus/prostate, and the entire abdominal cavity with beautiful golden-white light. . . . And then visualize the light flowing to the very tip of your spine, the tail bone, filling the buttocks with light, then moving down to the thighs, knees, calves, and ankles into the feet and out the tips of the toes. . . . And then let the same light flow into your shoulders, upper arms, elbows, forearms, wrists, and hands and out the fingertips. . . . Now that you have visualized this flow of light from head to toe and toe to head, you actually made it happen, since energy follows consciousness. Just open your awareness to a sense of a flow. . . ."

And then I would continue listing the kinds of perceptions that may occur, as outlined in the paragraph above. I deliver this guided imagery and warm-up exercise in a relaxing, somewhat hypnotic tone of voice. In my experience this is sufficient to "prime the pump" of even the most difficult first-time client.

If a client has worked in Inner Space before or is known to be psychically open, I do not waste many words. Invoking a higher-vibrational force field and a few words of guidance will usually be sufficient to help the client achieve a heightened state of awareness within one to three minutes.

When I am working with children, the induction is even less complicated: I silently invoke the light as I put my index and middle finger on their foreheads. Then I ask them to gently close their eyes and to tell me what colors they see coming from my fingers. In most cases, children report colors or other inner perceptions within 30 to 60 seconds, even when they prefer to keep their eyes open. In general, children seem to have fewer perceptual blocks than adults; thus they achieve more immediate access to Inner Space.

Chapter 10

Navigating Inner Space

Once the client has started to tap into Inner Space, things get a little more interesting for you, the healer, because it is your task to make sense of the reported perceptions and to guide the client's exploration in a useful direction. While Inner Space is principally unlimited in its possibilities, it is also somewhat lawful and understandable. This dual nature keeps the work interesting and, at times, challenging. As you gain experience, however, you will become quite comfortable in your role as pilot navigating Inner Space.

The Chakra System

In the realm of physical healing, a physician's examination may be guided by assessing the major organs (heart, liver, lungs, etc.), or by examining functional systems (such as the nervous or circulatory systems). Correspondingly, in the realm of energetic healing we tend to look either at the main energy centers, called chakras, or at energetic networks, of which the meridian system is most prominent. For our work, one of the most useful orientation maps is the ancient chakra system. (A later chapter will address meridian-based therapies.) We briefly mentioned the chakra system in the first part of this book. Now it is time to present a few more details.

There are seven major chakras within the physical body and numerous minor ones.[26] The major chakras are customarily numbered from one to seven, and have been given names and assigned colors in accordance with various traditions and teachings. Chakras may be likened to spinning cones or funnels of light. The second to sixth chakras can be described as pairs of cones extending from the spine out to the front and back of the body. The first and seventh chakras are more like single cones reaching downward and upward, respectively.

• The first, or "root" chakra, is located at the tip of the spine (the tailbone); its normal color is red. The glands most strongly affected by the first chakra are the adrenal glands. The anatomical areas most strongly affected are the spinal column and cord, (and therefore, in some respects, all parts of the body) as well as the anus and rectum.

• The second, or "navel" chakra, is located on the spine approximately an inch below the navel; its normal color is orange. The associated glands are the ovaries/testes. It affects the reproductive organs, bladder, uterus, kidneys, and the large intestine.

• The third, or "solar plexus" chakra, is located on the spine at the approximate level of the solar plexus (about halfway between the navel and the sternum); its normal color is yellow. The associated glands are the adrenal glands and the pancreas. It affects the liver, gall bladder, spleen, stomach, diaphragm, and the small intestine.

---

[26] Tradition and reference source can vary regarding details, terms, and assigned locations of the major chakras. We provide the following information as a guideline, not as absolute dogma.

• The fourth, or "heart" chakra, is located near the heart; its normal color is green. The associated gland is the thymus. It affects the heart, lungs, and esophagus, and the circulatory and respiratory systems.

• The fifth, or "throat" chakra, is located on the spine at the level of the Adam's apple; its normal color is blue. The associated glands are the thyroid and parathyroid. It affects the mouth, nose, ears, throat, tonsils, vocal cords, and the bronchial tract.

• The sixth, or "third eye" chakra, is located within the skull slightly above the nose and between the eyebrows; its normal color is indigo blue. The associated gland is the pituitary gland. It affects the frontal lobe, eyes, ears, nose, and sinuses.

• The seventh, or "crown" chakra, is located on top of the head where your find the fontanel; its normal color is violet. The associated gland is the pineal gland. It affects all parts of the brain, and therefore, in one way or another, every part of the body.

Note that the normal colors of the seven major chakras correspond to the colors of the rainbow, ranging from the lowest frequency, red, to the highest, violet. However, when clients perceive the chakras in Inner Space, they frequently report colors other than the ones we called "normal." This is not necessarily a reason for concern. We will discuss the various colors and their significance in a following chapter. Suffice it to say that any of the "healing" colors listed below is welcome in any of the chakras and should never be considered "out of place."

According to their function and frequency, the seven major chakras are customarily divided into lower (first to third) and higher (fifth to seventh) chakras, with the heart chakra having both a lower and a higher aspect. For optimal health on all levels, it is important that all chakras be open and spinning at their respective frequencies. Furthermore, the size and strength of each chakra should be in harmony and balance relative to the size and strength of the others.

Psychological Issues and the Major Chakras

Many books and schools of thought have put forward various theories regarding the relationship of psychological issues and the major chakras. While a fair degree of association is often apparent, we prefer our own observations to override any theoretical dogma. In general, we have found that many issues touch on more than one chakra at a time. Particularly when we are dealing with a complex system of crystallized energy blocks (to be discussed in a later chapter), the *a priori* assignment of a certain issue to a particular chakra becomes untenable. Thus, when it comes to making sense of the perceptions discovered in Inner Space, we would recommend avoiding rigid "cookbook" interpretations. Having said that, let us share some of the typical associations between "issues" and chakras that we have observed in our work.

The *first chakra* often carries issues connected with survival. It anchors us to the material plane, the physical world, and Mother Earth. The root chakra will respond particularly strongly when a person feels physically unsafe and threatened. Thus, it has also been called the "fight or flight" chakra.

The *second chakra* has been primarily associated with sexuality, procreation, and creativity (in conjunction with the fifth chakra). Our sexual drives and our sense of self as a man or a woman, as well as issues of guilt, shame, and sexual suppression, are often connected with the second chakra. Issues of power or the lack thereof can also be found in this area, again most often in conjunction with the fifth chakra.

The *third chakra* frequently reflects issues pertaining to emotional nurturing, support and connection. Many who have experienced a lack of nurturing, loneliness, disconnection, and emotional emptiness carry wounds or holes in their third chakras.

The *fourth chakra* is considered the primary portal through which the life force (or Light) connects with the body. While that is the function of all chakras, the heart chakra is, indeed, the "heart of it all." The issues of love of self or others, and the associated fears of vulnerability and disconnection from the source of love, dominate the heart chakra. The fourth chakra is also our main connecting point with our Higher Self and thus our main access to intuition, wisdom, and the Light from Source.

The *fifth chakra* tends to carry issues of guilt, shame, judgment of self and others, and an inability to accept and forgive self or others. In addition, the throat chakra harbors a sense of empowerment or lack thereof. If one is afraid to speak one's truth or feels overwhelmed, powerless, or victimized, the fifth chakra will inevitably be compromised.

The *sixth chakra* is more of a mental than an emotional chakra. It is primarily involved in thinking, perceiving, (psychic) vision, and related functions. If there is emotional scar tissue in the "third eye" chakra, it is often related to things one could not bear to see or hear, or negative thought forms that have taken root in the mind.

The *seventh chakra* is primarily a spiritual rather than an emotional chakra. The "crown" chakra is our portal to the "heavens," higher consciousness, and divine Light. It may be negatively affected by a thought of disconnection from the divine or by a crystallized energy block.

This delineation of the associations between chakras and psychological issues merely provides a guideline for orientation. It should not be interpreted in a prescriptive or "cookbook" fashion. Finally, here are two other general observations we have made in our work. (1) Very frequently there is an energetic connection between second chakra issues and fifth chakra issues. Thus, if one has found a major block in the second chakra, it is advisable to examine the fifth chakra as well. However, the reverse is not necessarily true, as there are throat chakra issues that may have little bearing on the second chakra. (2) Chakras that are closer together (e.g., third and fourth) are more likely to be simultaneously affected by the same psychological issue than chakras that are further apart (e.g., the first and seventh).

Chapter 11

Typical Perceptions in Inner Space

Inner Space is infinite in its possibilities and full of surprises. One of the greatest surprises may be that there are actually recognizable patterns that can be observed across individuals. Since most of our clients have never before explored Inner Space, and there is certainly nothing on TV or in the popular literature that would "educate" clients ahead of time on what to expect in Inner Space, the fact that there are typical perceptions that occur again and again is in itself remarkable. In this chapter we will list such typical perceptions and offer a guide to their interpretation.[27]

The most typical perceptions in Inner Space include: Colors; myriad images; perceptions of movement; physical sensations such as pain, burning, heat, cold, weight; inner tones; and feelings. We shall begin with the area of colors, as they are the foundation of much of our work. Of all the perceptions in Inner Space, colors tend to be the easiest to perceive, the easiest to describe, and the easiest to interpret.

Colors

We distinguish between "healing" colors and those that do not

---

[27] In order to benefit most from the information presented below, we suggest that you bookmark this page and temporarily turn to Chapter 12 which will introduce the distinction between "simple" and "crystallized energy blocks." This will help you to put some of the following information into a frame of reference. Then, when you return to Chapter 12 things will fall into place more easily.

carry a healing frequency. Whether a color is considered a healing color depends on a number of factors, particularly its hue and its secondary characteristics.

Healing colors typically have one or more of these attributes: They can be perceived as brilliant, iridescent, radiant, shiny, bright, vibrant, sparkly, alive, sunny, gentle, luminescent, or translucent.

Typical attributes that suggest that the observed color is *not* a healing color include murky, muddy, opaque, dark, dull, smoky, milky, chalky, flat, dense, "neon," "plastic," "shrill," fluorescent, cold, metallic, brassy, or "steely" qualities.

The different colors perceived in Inner Space can be subdivided into major and minor colors, according to the frequency with which they appear.

Major Colors

Red: Red is one of the most frequently observed colors in Inner Space. It is the natural color of the root (first) chakra. However, in 95 percent or more cases, red cannot be considered a healing color. If it is part of a *simple energy block*, it almost always denotes the feeling of anger or one of its cousins. If it is part of a *crystallized energy block*, red often denotes the energetic center of the crystallized energy block, without regard to the particular feeling that initially may have put such block in place. If we look at *physical tissue* from the perspective of Inner Space (such as an aching tooth or a post-surgical wound), red may suggest inflammation or irritation. Red is also often related to physical pain. Occasionally, the perception of red stands for fire or blood; in those cases, red is the entry point for a past life recall or the recall of a traumatic event from the present lifetime.

When you work with children for the first time, they may report seeing "a happy red" in their hearts because that is the color they traditionally associate with the heart. In that event, redirect them to seeing with their "inner" eye and tell them that the "inner" colors can be quite different from the ones perceived with our physical eyes.

In rare cases only do we count red as one of the healing colors. If we ask for healing light and red flows in as part of a rainbow of colors, it would certainly be welcomed. If the root chakra has been cleansed thoroughly, and the client is in need of some grounding or physically invigorating energies, a judicious use of red may be indicated. However, in contrast to some healers who advocate red for physical healing or invigoration, we almost always prefer to use other colors (such as a luminescent white) for such purposes.

Orange: Orange is the natural color of the naval (second) chakra. However, in the majority of cases we do not consider orange to be a healing color. Orange is often a companion color to red. If red, orange, and yellow are reported simultaneously, orange can be disregarded as a mixture of red and yellow; in such cases we attend primarily to the red, as yellow is more likely to be one of the healing colors and thus less of a reason for concern. When we find only orange, we ask the client to attempt to separate the orange into a red and a yellow. If that can be done easily, we pursue the red. If the color remains orange, however, we ask the client to probe the orange for associated feelings. Since the second chakra often carries sexual energies, probing in that direction may prove useful.

Pre-adolescent children and adolescents frequently show orange in their second chakras or in their extremities. While "raw" sexual energy is certainly part of the package of being human, orange is often not a very harmonious energy (and many kids struggle with their sexual feelings). In such cases, I suggest trying to blend the orange with violet or gold. Frequently, orange then turns into yellow or another color of higher frequency. This could be done without "exposing" the client to the possible significance of the orange vibration.

As with the color red, orange can be used as a healing color under some very limited circumstances. One such occasion is the introduction of orange into the second chakra, in the case of a client who has completely shut down the second chakra for a long time and needs some of that frequency to "jump-start" the navel chakra. But in most situations we prefer to work with higher-vibrational healing colors. For instance, we may suggest the blending of violet, yellow, or gold into the orange, if that was the predominant color of the second chakra. Orange found in any location other than the second chakra is probably not a healing color.

Yellow: Yellow is the natural color of the solar plexus (third) chakra. In many cases, yellow is a genuine healing color. Of all the healing colors, yellow is generally the weakest in potency. However, there are many situations in which yellow is exactly the right color for a specific need. Since the healing colors are an expression of a superior intelligence that knows best what is needed, we do not reject yellow if it presents itself in response to a request for a healing color. Occasionally, if progress appears slow, I will suggest boosting the yellow with some violet or gold.

In some cases and for some individuals, yellow may not be a healing color. In fact, some crystallized energy blocks produce energies that present as yellow. To distinguish one from the other, we need to pay attention to the context of yellow in the overall healing process. Furthermore, if the yellow appears flat, murky, opaque, or mustard-colored, or if the yellow borders on ocher or orange, some cleansing is clearly in order. Blending violet into the yellow will suffice in most cases. It is also possible that focusing on a "tainted" yellow may lead to an intensification of the murky qualities, which would then prompt further exploration.

Green: Green is the natural color of the heart (fourth) chakra. It is often perceived as an emerald or forest green. Green is always a healing color, provided it does not have any of the secondary characteristics that would suggest otherwise. Green is often the color of choice for healing of the heart chakra, for problems in the circulatory system, for wound healing, and for physical healing in general.

Should the green appear murky, "olivey," or like a military green, we will try to blend it with violet. Alternatively, we might seek to identify the brown or black components in the mix, which would then become the focus of our attention.

Blue: Blue is the natural color of the throat (fifth) chakra. It is often described as the blue one may see in the sky on a sunny day. Blue is almost invariably a healing color, with two possible but rare exceptions: if the blue has a metallic quality to it, or if it borders on black. In the latter scenario, I ask the blue to step aside, thus revealing the source of the black, which would then become our main concern. Blue is often the color of choice for the healing of typical throat chakra issues such as a sense of being overwhelmed, powerless, ashamed, guilty, or judgmental of self or others.

Golden-white: The golden-white light is often associated with the crown (seventh) chakra, but it is a powerful and welcome healing color wherever it presents itself. The golden-white light is also known as "the Light of the Christos"[28]. A true golden-white light is always a healing color, but on rare occasions a brassy metallic color associated with a crystallized energy block can be mistaken for a golden-white light.

The golden-white light is an excellent healing and sealing color for all purposes. It can also be employed as a tool during work in Inner Space. For instance, it can be used to encase, insulate, or highlight a crystallized energy block, or it could be applied like "WD-40" oil to loosen the grip of such a block and prepare it for easier removal.

Violet: The violet light, or Violet Flame, as it is also known, may be called the "universal cleansing agent." It is a powerful light that is most useful for the transformation and transmutation of lower-vibrational energies. It is truly the color of alchemy, "turning lead [gray] into gold [the Christos]." It is always a healing color and cannot be tainted or "faked" by crystallized energy blocks.

The colors belonging to the Violet Flame range from light violet to lavender and deep purple. In most cases, purple

---

[28] To avoid theological confusion, it may be opportune at this point to note that Jesus was a person who embodied the Christos, or Christ Light, in human form. However, the Christos is a universal and eternal energy and not limited to a specific embodiment or religious tradition.

is just a variation of violet and may be considered in the same way as violet. However, if the purple is bordering on red (magenta), it may actually be a mixture of red and violet. If the deep purple does not lighten up after a while, we will need to separate the colors by asking the violet to step aside so that we can explore the source of the red separately.

The presence of violet generally suggests that a transformation and transmutation of lower-vibrational energies is in process. Occasionally, if the violet light persists for an extraordinary length of time (circumstances and experience will tell you when that is the case), we suggest additional probing for the lower-vibrational energies that attracted the violet in the first place.

Violet is one of the colors typically associated with the crown chakra. It can also be found anywhere in the light body where there is a need for cleansing. Once the cleansing process is nearing completion, another healing color will often follow in the wake of the violet. If that is the case, one can be certain that the healing is well under way.

White: White may or may not be a healing color. When white appears in the company of gold, it is always welcome. The pure white light, without any gold, is also a healing color in its own right. It tends to energize and "shed light on things" and often comes in to seal in the healing work in a certain area. Frequently, white is the perfect color to mix into black or gray. However, unless the context leaves little room for doubt, it is important to ascertain that we are dealing with a bright, luminescent white and not a chalky, milky, or flat white. The latter is *not* a healing color and is often associated with crystallized energy blocks.

Gray: If the initial perception is of the color gray, it is often advisable to focus on the darkest spot in the gray and intensify it, so that it turns toward black. We would then treat it accordingly. If the initial perception is of a black color that gradually turns more into a gray, we consider this a good sign, as it suggests a "lightening up." If gray and black are perceived side by side, in most cases we focus on the black and disregard the gray.

Black: Black, as well as red, is one of the major indicators of lower-vibrational energies. It is never a healing color. It may indicate fear, shame, guilt, loss, depression, sadness, powerlessness, helplessness, "stale" anger, and other lower-vibrational energies. When clients perceive a lot of black within themselves, they may be disheartened or disgusted by their "darkness." In that case, it is useful to reframe this perception in a more positive light, by emphasizing that black indicates fertile ground for healing; it is grist for the mill. Metaphorically speaking, the black "coals" within can be turned into precious "diamonds" with the help of the healing light.[29]

Black, together with red, can often be found in or around crystallized energy blocks. In that case, black may carry little useful information. However, such spots may become an entry point for a past life recall or the recall of a traumatic event from the present lifetime.

Brown: Brown is most often a mixture of red and black. Depending on circumstances, the healer may choose to separate

---

[29] The natural process that turns carbon molecules from coal into diamonds is a fitting metaphor for the process of transformation and transmutation, or alchemy, which is at the heart of Psychoenergetic Healing.

brown into red and black and pursue each one separately, starting with the more intense of the two. Alternatively, we deal with brown as brown, looking for the deepest and densest spot in it, or seeking the spot from which the brown is emanating; then we proceed from there.

Pink: Pink is another one of the "tricky" colors requiring some astuteness on the part of the healer. When it presents itself as a soft, radiant pink, similar to that of rose quartz, it is a genuine healing color. It carries the vibration of love and can often be found in the heart chakra. In addition, pink is associated with healthy or healing tissue; it may be very helpful when physical healing is the issue.

On the other hand, pink may be a mixture of white and red. In that case, ask the client to separate it into its component colors and pursue the red first. Then, if necessary, check whether the white is of the milky/chalky variety or whether it is radiant, shiny, and translucent. In the latter case, we welcome the white as a healing color and give it more time to mix with the red. If the white shows questionable characteristics, we might need to address it as we did the red.

Pink may also present as "neon," "plastic," or "Pepto Bismal" pink, in which case it is clearly not a healing color. Most often, such pink does not separate well into red and white; we then deal with it as it presents itself.

Given the many faces of "pink," it is generally advisable to determine the nature of this color by inquiring about its secondary characteristics unless, of course, it is evident from the context what kind of pink we are dealing with.

Minor Colors

The following "minor" colors are reported far less often than the "major" colors listed above.

Indigo: Indigo is often associated with the third eye (sixth) chakra and is thus a healing color. However, it may also be a mixture of blue and black, in which case we again separate the two component colors and pursue the black, as usual. The context -- how we happened to encounter the indigo and at what stage in the process -- would provide some guidance as to the nature of this color.

Turquoise, aquamarine and other "mixed" colors should generally be counted among the healing colors. If such colors show themselves relatively often, they may indicate a person's "signature vibration"; you can interpret them as the main color of the client's Totality or Higher Self. A few clients have many such colors in their force fields but most do not report these "mixed" colors, at all.

Silver: Silver is *not* a healing color; it indicates a need for transformation. It is often associated with crystallized energy blocks and may prove at times to be rather resistant to change.

"**Clear**" is not really a color, but an energy that some clients report. It often fills an "empty" space. Blending the violet into it, or looking for the energetic center in the "empty" space, are two ways we deal with "clear."

For those readers who have little experience with working in Inner Space, the above list of major and minor colors and their various meanings may appear confusing and perhaps a bit daunting. With a little patience, however, working with colors will prove a reliable and useful tool for your transformational work. If you pay scrupulous attention to the context and secondary characteristics of the colors, you will learn to work with the colors with great effectiveness.

Next, we will discuss some of the other typical perceptions that arise in Inner Space.

Images

Inner Space can present myriad visual perceptions that may all be called "images." For purposes of instruction, we have broken down these images into several somewhat arbitrary categories that we labeled geometric shapes, geometric patterns, technical images, directional images, figures and animals, and bizarre images. All these images indicate the presence of crystallized energy blocks.

An altogether different class of images includes perceptions of the physical body from within Inner Space, present or past-life images, and miscellaneous visions (visions of outer space, visions of the future, spiritual visions, etc.). Such imagery is generally very rich in useful information and should be treated quite differently from the confusing mirages produced by crystallized energy blocks.

Again, as in dealing with colors, the range of images perceived in Inner Space requires some astuteness and experience on the part of the healer as he or she separates the wheat from the chaff. The following guidelines will give you a head start in your learning process.

Geometric shapes: This category includes shapes of triangles, squares, diamonds (such as the ones found on a deck of cards), cubes, spheres, boxes, tubes, cones, belts, rings, circles, wheels, stars, shields, etc. Any abstract, geometric shape found in Inner Space suggests a crystallized energy block -- with the possible exception of pyramids, and shapes perceived as part of a spiritual or "outer space" vision. To dissolve such blocks we try to penetrate the energetic center of the shape, which is often close to its geometric center.

Geometric patterns: Two- or three-dimensional geometric patterns (lattices, white lace, line patterns, plaid, etc.) are similar in nature to the shapes mentioned above, with the major difference that they tend to lack a clearly identifiable center. They may be quite distracting and "annoying." Their presence suggests that we are dealing with peripheral layers and that there is still a way to go before we have reached the energetic center of the energy block.

Technical images: The range of technical images perceived in Inner Space is virtually unlimited and often quite bizarre. One client reported seeing an airport or a railroad station in her knees, another saw a boiler room with elaborate ductwork in her liver, others reported switchboards, engines, and many other technical, futuristic, or industrial images. Occasionally, such imagery may have some symbolic meaning. For the most part, however, we disregard the details and treat the perception as a mirage or distraction created by a crystallized energy block.

Directional images: Generally more productive than geometric patterns or technical images are images that tend to give a direction to our exploration in Inner Space. Typical perceptions in this category may be hallways, staircases, doors, tunnels, funnels, chutes, holes, alleys, and so on. In most instances we direct the client to go into the tunnel, through the door, down the staircase, etc. Very often this will lead us to another place or image and, ultimately, closer to the energetic center of the crystallized block.

Figures and animals: There are four classes of figures, each with a slightly different significance. The first class are *figures that appear in groups*, often milling about chaotically. Among them are Packman-like figures, "gray fuzzies," cartoon-like figures, ET-like figures, or simply a group of faceless "people." Figures in this category tend to be found at the periphery of crystallized energy blocks; thus, they carry relatively little charge and strength. Using a sound, or transformational light, usually takes care of these perceptions.

The second class we call *guardian figures,* because they are part of the "defense system" of a crystallized energy block. Their task is to guard the center of such a block from discovery and transformation, usually by assuming a frightening appearance and demeanor. Fiery dragons, growling lions or wolves, scary masks, spiders, snakes, or gargoyles are among the guardian figures most often reported. We deal with such figures by directing the client to go into "the belly of the beast," either through the eyes or the mouth, and to find the spot within the figure that holds the greatest charge. This is likely to take us a significant step closer to the center of the crystallized energy block.

The third class includes *"entities"* such as wizards, witches, "Tasmanian devils," magicians, witch doctors, demons, goblins, tricksters, or other humanoid or animal-like figures. They appear to be alive and to have wills of their own, which are expressed in either words, thoughts, or gestures. Typically, they display an "attitude" through laughter, ridicule, or mockery. If they feel cornered they may turn to evasion, pleading, or other maneuvers. Figures of this kind are often a bit testy and challenging. While they may protest that they are only there to "help" or "teach," do not fall for their attempts to deceive you!

We normally try to engage such "entities" in dialogue, but they may choose not to answer, in which case, we move ahead with the "eviction proceedings." If they are willing to enter into a dialogue, we may ask what their purpose is, whether they are serving the Light, how long they have been with the client, or whether they are willing to go into the Light. The "entity" may or may not be willing to answer honestly, and may or may not be willing to step into the Light. Occasionally, a long and -- at times -- informative exchange may ensue.

Generally, it is a good idea to honor the figure, thank it for its services, surround it with love and light, and send it on its way. Invoking the help of Archangel Michael and/or the Violet Flame may be useful at that point. If the figure is hanging on, we obviously need to explore the source of its power supply, including any ambivalence and attachment on the part of the client. Once that has been accomplished, the lifting off should occur more easily.

In the fourth category are *figures of humans that carry a symbolic meaning.* For instance, a woman may perceive a dead baby in her womb; this may be related to issues connected with an abortion, a miscarriage, or a "lost twin." An image of a child huddling in a corner, protecting his face, may be related to a history of abuse from either the present or a past lifetime. In most cases, we would surround such a human figure with healing light and observe the response. In the case of the dead baby, for instance, the image may transform or disappear as we uncover the emotional story behind the image. In the case of the child huddling in a corner, the image may come to life slowly, and the child may give up his protective posture and scared expression. We would also ask the child to describe what frightened him so. We would then process the associated images or memories, and we would comfort and reassure him that his feelings are understood and that he can feel safe now. In other words, we would deal with him as a person within a person. As the healing nears completion the image is likely to change, for instance into that of a happy and carefree child. In that case, our goal is not to dissolve or eliminate the figure but to heal, integrate, and embrace the symbolic "child within."

Bizarre images: As with dream imagery, the range of bizarre images that may occur in Inner Space is virtually unlimited. Among this group of images there are again two classes. The first class includes utterly bizarre images that carry little, if any, meaning. These images may be rather elaborate and involved. Their sole purpose is to confuse and distract from the healing process; they are part of the smoke screen generated by deeply entrenched crystallized energy blocks. A client who reports many such mirages could be highly defended, ambivalent, or otherwise stuck. Clients who smoke, have a poor diet, or use many medications such as pain killers are more likely to report imagery of this kind.[30]

---

[30] This observation may lend support to the notion of "energy toxins" as proposed in Thought Field Therapy and other meridian-based therapies.

The second class of bizarre images can be found more frequently and can be dealt with more productively. These include images of bones, needles, nails, sponges, knots, spools, coals, fire, cauldrons, ponds, caves, knives, spears, fists, octopus-like tentacles, "hot" electric wires with sparks, skeletons, and many similarly bizarre perceptions. Depending on the circumstances, we might suggest going into the tip of the needle or knife, the center of the knot or coal, or the bottom of the pond. Once the client has made contact with the energetic center of the perception -- and that may require going through a number of layers -- the transformation of the crystallized block can proceed more easily.

Occasionally, some of the images we classified as "bizarre" may actually have a very straightforward meaning. A knife or spear may point to a past life in which such weaponry was used to inflict injury or death. Or the perception of fire may lead to an awareness of a traumatic experience that occurred in the current or a past lifetime. Thus, we have to stay open to the possibility that "sometimes a cigar is just a cigar."

Shape shifting: In the context of bizarre imagery, we should mention a phenomenon we call "shape shifting." This happens when one strange or bizarre image turns into another and another and another. Shape shifting is a clear indication of a crystallized energy block that is using distraction and confusion as its means of defense.

Movements

Movement, or lack thereof, is another important indicator that helps us to navigate Inner Space. Here are some typical ways that movement may be described:

Stagnation: Stagnation means the absence of movement of any kind. This tends to signify a "dead" energy space, numbness, or an energy block that has not been activated yet. We would try to mix a transformative color, such as a violet, into a stagnant energy in order to bring the "dead" energy to life. If the stagnation results from numbness put into place by the client, having the client affirm that he or she now chooses to become aware of the information contained in the block may prove helpful.

Side-to-side drifting: Clients may perceive stripes, bands, or clouds moving from one side of the "visual field" to the other. In most cases, these perceptions indicate the presence of disharmonious energies. Although some of these perceptions may include healing colors, the side-to-side drifting of distinct shapes would still suggest that more cleansing is in order.

Swirling and spinning: Any movement around an energetic center point is a welcome sign that we have tapped into a vortex of energy. If this energy is of the healing variety, such as a spinning vortex of violet light, we allow it to run its course and invite it to go wherever it needs to go. If the context or colors suggest the presence of an energetic block, we would encourage the client to enter into the center of the perceived movement, which may then lead straight to the heart of the energetic block.

Pulsating, vibrating, trembling, and contracting: Perceptions of this kind clearly indicate the presence of a crystallized energy block. Nevertheless, a healer would welcome the report of such movement for the same reason that a hawk likes a mouse to move: It makes it easier to zero in on the target. As usual, we would guide the client to go to the very center of the perceived movement, which would soon guide us to the heart of the crystallized energy block.

Physical Sensations

When clients enter into Inner Space, they may experience any number of physical sensations that may be very real and tangible in nature. Here are some of the typical physical sensations experienced by our clients:

Warmth and tingling: At the beginning of a session, or following the removal of an energetic block, clients may report warmth or tingling. This suggest the inflow of light into areas previously undersupplied. We would encourage the client to allow the warmth or tingling to expand and to spread throughout the affected area, or even the whole body.

Floating: This is one of those perceptions that can have widely different meanings. Sometimes floating is the initial sensation, which signifies that the client is entering into another frequency (such as a trip into "outer space" or other dimensions). This is most likely the meaning of "floating" if it follows in the wake of a significant energetic shift. In that case, we would encourage the client to go along with the floating and to drift wherever it may take him or her.

Another situation altogether occurs when floating indicates that the client is leaving his or her body because of a dissociative response to a traumatic experience. In a case like that, we would ask the client to describe in detail what is happening in the scene. Ultimately, after some preparatory work, we would encourage the client to reenter his or her body as the events unfold. Reversing the dissociation has proven to be a crucial step in the healing process.

Lightness or heaviness: Lightness of the whole body may be a precursor to floating. However, when the sensation of lightness is limited to a body part (such as an arm or leg) it tends to suggest the presence of an energy block. In that case, we might ask for a more detailed description of the body part's color, the focal point of the lightness, where it begins, etc.

Similarly, "heaviness" of a body part most often indicates an energetic block. In that event, we would ask the client to increase the sense of heaviness and then to perceive in greater detail the spot that appears heaviest.

Weight: We listed "weight" as a category separate from "heaviness." "Weight" pertains to the perception of a heavy weight, such as a boulder, or similar pressure put on one's body. In some cases this sensation may have little significance beyond indicating the presence of an energetic block; in other cases it may serve as an entry point for the recall of a traumatic event -- most often from a past life -- when such weight was indeed put on the person's body. Two typical examples of past-life memories that were prompted by the intense experience of weight are being crushed by a boulder or buried under a horse in battle.

Shrinking or ballooning of the body: If a client reports a disproportionate shrinking or ballooning of the entire body or, more often, of parts of the body, we can assume the presence of a crystallized energy block.

Twitches, spasms, jerking, convulsing, restless legs: This category includes involuntary body movements ranging from slight twitches to massive convulsions.[31] In all cases you may assume the presence on a crystallized energy block. If the spasm becomes the focus of attention, we would try to unravel the energetic block through that focal point. If it is merely a distraction attempt arising in response to our probing into an energetic block, we would be inclined to ignore the involuntary movements and pursue our initial line of inquiry.

Pain: The physical pain that some clients may experience from energetic blockage can be rather severe.[32] They may describe their pain as cramping, stabbing, burning or in any other way that pain may manifest. It is important not to be intimidated by such events, as the pain may be no more than a means of defense for crystallized energy blocks. Most pain can be resolved in minutes. The healer should reassure the client and encourage him or her to enter the focal point where the

---

[31] If a client is convulsing, or thrashing from side to side, it may be a little frightening to watch, particularly if it happens for the first time. One may feel reminded of popular movies depicting states of "demonic possession." It is, however, not a reason for concern, if the healer remains calm and centered in the Light. Simply encourage the client to keep breathing the Light, while you do the same.

[32] It is important to note, however, that pain induced by energetic blocks is not a phenomenon limited to working in Inner Space. Headaches, stomachaches, abdominal cramping, etc., may occur without any "physical" reason. In fact, as "all is energy," we posit that *all* pain is the result of an energetic disturbance, regardless of the presence or absence of any identifiable physical "cause."

pain seems most intense. Once the barrier of awareness has been penetrated, healing energy can flow into the painful spot and, in all likelihood, the pain will subside instantaneously. If that is not the case, the pain may be a harbinger of a deeper trauma that is still waiting to be uncovered. One client, for instance, experienced severe headaches in our first session that would not diminish easily until she discovered a history of being tortured with a head iron in medieval times. However, in most cases, the pain, regardless of intensity, is of short duration only.[33]

Heat and burning: In contrast to the "warmth" discussed previously, "heat" tends to be more intense, sharper, more focused, and less pleasant. In a few instances, the sensation of heat or burning may approach the intensity of a cigarette burning one's skin. Again, we would focus the client's attention on the hottest, most intense spot. In the majority of cases, this would lead us closer to the energetic center of the block. Occasionally, pursuing the heat may become the entry point for a past-life recall. For example, the physical sensation of heat, or the visual appearance of fire (see above), was the initial perception that brought several of our clients in touch with memories of being burnt on the stake.

"Hot flashes," chills, and shivering: Some clients, and this is not limited to menopausal women, may experience intense "hot flashes" and sweating, or chills and trembling and shiver-

---

[33] Sometimes a client presents with aches or pains which have nothing to do with working in Inner Space, such as a sprained ankle or a day-old headache. In most cases these pains can be easily remedied. We will talk more about this in Chapter 17.

ing. Some have asked for a blanket in the heat of summer. We attribute most of these fluctuations in body temperature to an imbalance in the autonomic nervous system.[34] Such temperature fluctuations typically indicate the presence of a crystallized energy block. As usual, we would encourage the client to enter into the hottest or coldest spot in the body and then to describe its color, shape, texture, or movement in greater detail.

Tightness and tension: Muscular tension, or a sense of tightness anywhere in the body, are typical physical sensations when working in Inner Space. Such sensations may point to either simple or crystallized energy blocks. In any event, we would direct the client to intensify the tension or tightness and then to penetrate its center. Simply focusing attention on that particular area may cause the tightness or tension to dissolve -- even as the client attempts to intensify it. We would take such an event as a sign that healing is already in progress.

Coughing, choking, and breathing difficulties: Coughing is one of the most frequent physical responses encountered in our work. It is a clear indication of either a simple or a crystallized energy block in the throat chakra (and sometimes also in the chest area). When the tightness in the throat intensifies, there may be a sense of choking or strangulation. Breathing difficulties may also become quite intense. Again, we are faced with two possible meanings: either the sensations are generated by an energetic block, or they are the first step toward un-

[34] A special case are "hot flashes" arising from the stirring of the kundalini energy, a phenomenon we will discuss in Chapter 21.

covering a history of strangulation, asphyxiation, smoke inhalation, drowning, or similar traumatic experiences.

Nausea: Nausea indicates without exception the presence of an energetic block, typically in the third chakra. So far, two of my clients have actually vomited (in the bathroom, fortunately), so I make sure to have a container handy for emergencies. Such provision allows me to ask the client to intensify the nausea without fear of consequences.

While nausea is not uncommon, actual vomiting is very rare. I mention this possibility for two reasons: to illustrate that working with energies is not something that "only happens in your mind," and to let fellow practitioners know that there is no reason for alarm in the rare event that a client may respond with vomiting.

Dizziness or spinning: Sensations of dizziness, spinning, or of losing the ground under one's feet comprise another class of physical sensations that clients occasionally experience. In most cases we would look for evidence of a crystallized energy block generating such sensations.

Following the opening of the third eye or sixth chakra clients may encounter a temporary increase of dizziness. A simple remedy for such a symptom is to hand the client a piece of paper depicting the full spectrum of rainbow colors and to have the client gaze repeatedly at the rainbow colors whenever he or she experiences dizziness.

Emptiness and numbness: Emptiness and numbness suggest the lack of energy or awareness in a certain area of the energy body, most often in conjunction with a crystallized energy block. Even though the client describes the space as empty, I routinely direct the client to the spot that seems "most empty." Inevitably, what appeared to be empty, void, or hollow proves not to be so at all. There is always some information contained in or hidden by the "empty" spot.

Sexual sensations: Primarily when they are working on the second chakra, some clients may experience sexual sensations. We allow such sensations and, at times, even encourage them. In any event, we ask for details regarding the colors and other characteristics of the sexual energies and most likely will suggest a blending with violet, gold or another appropriate healing color.

Clients with a history of sexual abuse are often afraid of their sexual energies because they are so intertwined with painful emotions such as shame, guilt, and fear. Consequently, they tend to block their experience of the sexual energies in order to avoid the associated negative feelings. In such cases, to experience their sexual energies without contamination, in the safety of a higher-vibrational energy field, may prove very healing indeed.

Extreme tiredness or drifting off: Some clients experience spells of extreme tiredness and may even fall asleep. While sleeping can be healing and productive under certain conditions, when clients doze off repeatedly, or drift off into "lala land," productive work may become almost impossible. One or two clients of mine have gotten into such a deep state of unconsciousness that I had to touch them and call their names repeatedly to bring them back to waking consciousness. A sudden attack of tiredness or the inability to stay awake and focused, indicates the presence of a crystallized energy block and presents one of the greatest challenges a healer can encounter. The only good thing that can be said about this phenomenon is that it occurs relatively rarely.

Tones

A few individuals are more auditory than visual and respond better to perceptions of tones. Sound is just another expression of energy; we approach it as we do colors. However, we do not have as extensive and specific a vocabulary to describe tones, as we have to describe colors. This makes it more difficult for the client to communicate the perceptions discovered in Inner Space and more difficult for the healer to give confident guidance. Ultimately, it does not matter whether we interpret the frequencies as colors or as tones. Let your client's preference guide you. Asking for a healing tone to permeate the client's body can be very helpful, either as an adjunct modality or as the main healing technique with a particular client.[35]

Feelings

The emotions clients discover in this line of work encompass the full range of human experience, from the deepest despair and agony to the highest ecstasy and bliss. The level of emotional intensity varies, of course, with the temperament of the client and the issue at hand. Not all sessions are highly emotional nor is it always necessary for intense emotions to arise in order for a healing to take place. As a healer, however, you

[35] We will discuss the use of sound as a healing tool in Chapter 14.

must not be afraid of intense expressions of emotions, uncontrollable sobbing, rivers of tears, and the occasional scream.

Emotions are what they are; they require little translation or interpretation -- with one exception. There are what we call "decoy" emotions, notably sadness and related feelings, which may be a part of a system of defense organized around a crystallized energy block. If a client starts feeling sad all of a sudden, just when we are making headway in our probing of a crystallized energy block, we encourage the client to move right through the layer of sadness. Often, the sadness or related emotion disappears as quickly as it arose. In that case, the "decoy" emotion was a smoke screen, arising to distract and confuse the client, and it is important for the healer not to fall for the trick.

Chapter 12

Simple and Crystallized Energy Blocks

Up to this point, we have made many references to simple and crystallized energy blocks. Now we can turn our attention to a thorough definition.

Simple Energy Blocks

Simple energy blocks are barriers to awareness that the individual created to avoid emotions and feelings that appeared too painful, frightening, overwhelming, or unpleasant. You can think of these barriers as "Ziploc bags" containing unprocessed emotions and experiences. On the energetic level such barriers of awareness "seal in" the affect and "freeze" it in time; it remains dormant until some event or circumstance dissolves or breaks through the barriers and creates an energetic shift.

One of the basic metaphysical laws in effect in this corner of the universe is the law of free will. All higher-vibrational energies honor and respect our free-will choices. If we put barriers in place that say, in effect, "I don't want to know or feel my feelings," the Light will oblige. Such barriers then stop the free flow of healing energies, thus preserving the energetic disturbance indefinitely.[36] As we are the ones who put those barriers in place, we are also the ones who hold the key to dissolving them. In general, it is necessary to become aware

[36] "Time" does not heal any wounds -- "energy" does!

of the information contained in a block. "You have to feel it in order to heal it."[37]

Crystallized Energy Blocks

Crystallized energy blocks are configurations of disharmonious energies that appear to have developed a "will" of their own. There are many conditions under which an energy block may become crystallized. Often, such blocks develop when there has been a past- or present-life trauma of great strength or duration, but many other factors (such as toxic substances, thoughts, or habits) may also contribute to the development of crystallized blocks.

Since these blocks appear to have a "will" of their own, they may pose a significant challenge to the healer who is trying to restore a more harmonious flow of energies. Typically, crystallized blocks will try to resist or evade the influx of healing light. They can employ a host of techniques to prevent their discovery or removal, just the way viruses or parasites do. Their defense efforts will present the healer with anything from minor obstacles to major headaches, depending on various factors we will discuss later. These blocks may be limited to one area only, or they may have developed an elaborate system of "pipelines" that provide the fuel for manifestations of energetic blocks throughout the body.

It is important to understand that such blocks are ultimately the (unconscious) creation of the individual; they are not some separate entity or evil force. The essence of these

[37] Exceptions to this rule of thumb may include work with children, absentee healing on others, and some cases of "physical" healing.

blocks is based on separation from the Light. To think of them as separate from us or adversarial to ourselves only serves to reinforce such blocks ("What you resist persists"). This realization is crucial to our understanding of the healing process. It is more in alignment with the fundamental principles of our work than fear-based concepts that embrace notions of evil spirits, hostile entities, or possession by outside forces.[38]

How to Distinguish Between Simple and Crystallized Energy Blocks

Distinguishing one kind of block from another is relatively easy but, as with everything occurring in Inner Space, the distinction is not entirely black and white. *Simple energy blocks* are comparatively uncomplicated structures that primarily contain raw emotional information rather than elaborate defense systems or nonsensical "garbage." The emotional information contained in simple blocks is relatively close to the surface and may gush out once we have unsealed the "Ziploc bag." There are few obstacles to uncovering the emotional information beyond the fear, discomfort, shame, guilt, and so on that prompted the person to seal away the emotional experience in the first place. All we need to do is dismantle the barriers to awareness and the healing can proceed instantaneously.

Crystallized energy blocks may or may not contain useful emotional information (below, we distinguish between

---

[38] We do not argue for or against the validity of such ideas. However, the need to "defend" the self from forces "out there" is fear-based and lower-vibrational in nature; it can ultimately create the very experience we wish to defend ourselves against. As a rule, as co-creators of our world we are prone to draw to us the very things we fear the most.

"productive" and "unproductive" varieties). As energies that have developed something like a "will" of their own, these blocks are primarily invested in self-preservation. Which strategies a particular block employs to resist healing and transformation depends on the nature of the block and its level of sophistication.

We described many of the telltale signs of crystallized energy blocks in the previous chapter. Here is an abridged list of the manifestations that we mentioned earlier: Geometric shapes and patterns; technical images; directional images, bizarre images, and images of figures and animals; shape shifting; pulsations; emptiness; dizziness; nausea; tightness; choking; "hot flashes" and chills; pain; burning; weight; heaviness; ballooning; spasms; extreme tiredness; colors with smoky, milky, chalky, "neon," "plastic," "shrill," metallic, fluorescent, cold, silvery, or "steely" qualities.

If all of the above strikes you as a lot of cumbersome, hard-to-remember information, let us assure you that with experience you will simply know what kind of energy block you are dealing with and what to do about it. Remember when you learned to drive a car? You had to learn a lot of technical jargon that you may or may not remember now. Nevertheless, chances are that you are a better driver now than when you were first learning all the details in your driver's ed class. Finding your way through Inner Space is another skill you can master with equal success.

How to Discover Energetic Blocks

When we look into outer space on a starry night, we are more likely to focus on the moon, stars, and planets than on the darkness of the void. Similarly, when we look into Inner Space, we are more likely to focus on a prominent energetic block than on a sea of healing colors. In fact, healing light is most often characterized by the presence of a continuous flow without a clearly defined form or focus. Thus, looking for a focus of awareness in Inner Space is almost synonymous with searching for energetic blocks.

Let us assume that you have set up a higher-vibrational energy field, guided the client into Inner Space, and established some sense of a flow within. The next step is to ask the client to report any and all observations of Inner Space phenomena without censure or editing. You will also ask the client for a focus of awareness.

If there is no stable awareness of a healing light yet, you can put two fingers on the client's Third Eye and ask what colors are flowing from your fingertips. Sometimes the answer is "red" or "black." These, of course, are not colors that would flow from the healer's fingertips, but they are nevertheless useful starting points for the healing work.

If the answer indicates the presence of a healing color, ask the client to allow that light to expand throughout the body. Then suggest that the client take his or her inner sight on a tour through the body to check for any areas that are resistant to such light. You can ask whether the healing color is flowing easily into the arms, hands, legs, and feet, up and down the spine, etc. If the client discovers an area that is less open to the healing light, focus on that area and ask for details.

If the client observes anything beyond healing colors, *pursue that focus of awareness* (i.e., the greatest pain, strongest heat, heaviest weight, greatest discomfort, darkest color, etc.) This is the direction you will follow in most cases. However, crystallized energy blocks sometimes try to distract attention by intensifying the client's discomfort. Occasionally, you may choose to ignore such distractions in order to search for the root cause, instead. But usually you will pursue the focus of awareness as it arises. In the following paragraphs, we will describe five techniques you may use to sharpen and intensify such focus.

(1) If the client reports only a faint perception, encourage him or her to intensify that perception through "breathing into it," putting his/her awareness into it, looking at it through a "magnifying glass," "pouring oil into the fire," making the weight heavier, intensifying the pain, etc. Remember: "Energy follows consciousness," and "Where there is more light, there is more shadow." Thus, a focused awareness tends to result in a clearer perception of any blocks that may exist.

(2) Occasionally, you may perceive a block through observation, intuition, or empathy. For instance, you or your client may start coughing the moment you enter into Inner Space. This would suggest, of course, that there are throat chakra issues to be explored. Or you can hook up with your client empathically and your find heart starting to ache. Then you might choose to bring the client's attention to the heart chakra. Trust such perceptions and, if prompted by your inner guidance, suggest that that area become the focus of your client's attention.

(3) If you know beforehand what the issue is -- from talking with the client or from the problem or history the client presented -- you may suggest that he or she focus on the chakras that tend to be associated with such issue. For instance, suppose a client feels guilty about a sexual indiscretion. Under these circumstances you can safely assume that the chakras affected by these issues include at least the second (sexuality)

and fifth (judgment). Either chakra would be a good place to begin your investigations.

(4) If you suspect the presence of certain issues that your client may or may not be aware of, you can ask an open-ended test question and watch for an energetic response. If you suspect, for instance, that a child client is uncomfortable in school, you might ask the child to look for a resonance within while you bring up that issue: "Look around your body and tell me where you notice a response when you think about 'school'."

(5) If your client enters Inner Space and cannot find an immediate or clear focus of awareness, point out that his or her inner guidance might be able to suggest a focal or entry point for the work. In response, your client may experience a twitching, discomfort, a visual image, or some other manifestation that indicates where his or her attention is going. You can also ask for such inner guidance yourself and use the information that arises to direct your client's attention.

Once a focus of awareness has been established, ask for details: colors and their quality; shapes and forms; texture; size or depth; weight; heat or cold; solid, liquid, or gaseous consistency; movement, or lack thereof; or whatever else seems important. This information gathering process helps (a) to further intensify the focus of awareness and (b) to determine the nature of the energetic block.[39] It is not necessary to inquire about each and every aspect of the block your client is

---

[39] Obviously, if the information contained in the block is close to the surface (i.e., you encounter a strong emotional or physical response, or clear images from this or a past life), the descriptive details of the block are less important.

observing. Ask just enough questions to move the process along and to determine whether you are dealing with a simple or a crystallized energy block. *This is the first major junction on our decision-making tree.*

Chapter 13

How to Deal with Energy Blocks

How to Deal With Simple Energy Blocks

Let us assume that you have encountered what appears to be a simple energy block. Ask your client to stay focused on that block and to allow an awareness of the thoughts, feelings, or images contained in the block to emerge. If no such awareness immediately arises, ask your client to focus on the energetic center of the block (e.g., "Go to where it is darkest or densest") and to enter that center. Then suggest that the client ask his or her inner guidance for help. If nothing is forthcoming, there are a number of techniques that may help your client overcome the barriers to awareness:

(1) You may ask for more details, such as the features listed above (colors and their quality; shapes and forms; texture; size; weight; heat or cold; solid, liquid, or gaseous consistency; movement or lack thereof, etc.). Then pursue whatever arises (e.g., "go into the center of the circle," "make the weight heavier," "sink into the gray liquid," and so on). This line of inquiry may ultimately result in your client's discovery of the emotional information stored in the block.

(2) You may ask the client, "In response to the following question, give me a number, the first number that comes to mind. How old is that [dark/heavy/painful, etc.] spot?" Upon

hearing a number (e.g., "seven"[40]), ask: "What sounds most like it: Seven months, seven years, when you were seven, or seven lifetimes ago?" Then ask the client to go to the time and place that come up when thinking of the time indicated. If necessary, ask additional questions about that scene (e.g., time of the year, day or night, indoors or out, alone or with others, attire, etc.) until a clearer focus develops.

(3) Another approach is to list a number of feelings (e.g., shame, guilt, loss, helplessness, hopelessness, depression, loneliness, greed, anger, fear, emptiness, etc.) and ask your client to check for an inner response. Often there is an energetic or emotional response to one or more of the feelings mentioned, which then serves as a point of departure for further exploration.

(4) If a client has zeroed in on a block in his or her body but has not yet been able to uncover the information contained in it, you could hold your hand above that spot and send focused energy into it. "Where there is more light, there is more shadow" -- so this technique may sharpen the client's awareness.

Once a sufficient degree of awareness has been established, ask the client to accept without judgment all feelings and thoughts that come up. If necessary, suggest that your client intensify the feeling for a moment (e.g., "let the sadness fill your whole body," or "allow yourself to get really mad").

---

[40] We have noticed that age seven figures prominently in many clients' lives. Astrologically, a child experiences his or her first Saturn square (i.e., Saturn in the heavens aspecting the child's natal Saturn at a 90 degree angle) at that age, which often brings with it experiences of fear, loss, separation, loneliness, rejection, and a first encounter with responsibilities that foster maturity.

At this point it is essential for the healer to maintain a soothing and supportive manner. New clients may need reassurance that their intensified suffering will be brief and that they can count on relief.

When you sense that your client has connected with the emotion he or she had been avoiding, suggest that the client open him- or herself to a healing radiance. Often it is useful to ask what healing color(s) may come to the client "automatically" and whether the color or feeling in the block and the healing color(s) can mix easily. If the client has a sense of a healing color offering itself, encourage the client to open him- or herself to the light and to ask for healing and transformation. Ask your client to tell you when all of the block seems to have been dissolved. It may also be useful to ask what healing color is present in the target area when your client indicates that the transformation is complete. If the block and the healing colors stopped mixing before the lower-vibrational energy has been absorbed completely, or the colors do not blend at all ("like oil and water"), further exploration is indicated.

If only a portion of the block can be transformed, the client may need to go back into the block to unearth additional information. For instance, if there is a red color containing anger at both someone else *and* the self, both may need to be acknowledged before all the red can be dissolved.

If the energetic block stems from a traumatic experience, either from the current or a past life, you may choose to enter that time and space and heal it on the higher planes (more about that later). Once the past has been healed, its energetic residue in the client's light body can be transformed more easily.

At times a client cannot let go of his or her judgment of a feeling or an action. Judgment interferes with healing, so you will need to explore the barriers to healing in greater detail. Feelings of guilt and a deep sense of unworthiness are frequent obstacles to a client's acceptance of the healing light. Ask your client, "Where in your body is the space that holds this sense of guilt [or unworthiness or whatever it may be]?" Then pursue that focus as you would any other.

Occasionally, you may need to dig a little deeper. For example, a mother leaves her family to live with a lover. Years later she still carries deep guilt and remorse about "abandoning" her children. The simple suggestion that she release her guilt feelings and forgive herself may not suffice. Instead, we may need to enter into an exploration of past-life connections between all the players in order to understand more fully the karmic story behind the drama. Depending on the circumstances, it may also be helpful to initiate a dialogue with a being of Light or the Higher Selves of your client and of the person(s) "offended." Once the karmic background is better understood, you can proceed with healing on the higher planes (more about that in Chapter 17 & 18). Finally, the client will be able to forgive him- or herself and you can proceed with the healing of the block that prompted this line of probing.

As you may recall from our discussion of the healing colors, violet (or purple) is the universal cleansing agent. The continued presence of violet/purple indicates that the active transformation process is still occurring. Under these circumstances, it is best to give the process more time. Then ask your client which other color(s) follow in the wake of the violet once it has completed its cleanup work. If the violet does not seem to make the expected progress, you may need to take another look at whatever is attracting the persistent presence of violet. At that point, further exploration and the use of sound (which we will discuss later) could be in order.

If there seems to be no trace left of the simple energy block, and the space where the block was first observed is filled with healing colors, the healing of that particular issue is well underway. If time permits, you then move on to another block -- one that may reveal itself only after the initial block has been healed.

How to Deal With Crystallized Energy Blocks

Distinguishing Between "Productive" and "Unproductive" Blocks

We can distinguish between two kinds of crystallized energy blocks: Those that should be explored from within the block (the "productive" variety) and those that should simply be removed or dissolved (the "unproductive" variety). *This is the second major junction on our decision-making tree.*

Experience, intuition, and guidance from the healer's Higher Self and other beings of Light are useful in helping one negotiate the myriad manifestations of crystallized energy that one may encounter in Inner Space. The following guidelines will give you a fairly good idea of what you may encounter, but sometimes only trial and error will indicate which way to go.

Blocks of the "unproductive" variety tend to be emotionally relatively neutral (no intense feelings, no discomfort or fear associated with them), and more abstract or unstructured in appearance (e.g., worms, spaghetti, cubes, sponges, clouds, milky white or silvery colors, etc.). In contrast to the way we approach all other energy blocks, there is little to be gained by entering a block of the "unproductive" variety. Either the block is inaccessible, or it leads into a haze of confusion, or it could be easily removed without close scrutiny and without wasted time. A focused application of sound or violet light or the help of Archangel Michael may be sufficient to dissolve such blocks. Only if the blocks do not dissolve will you need to pursue further exploration.

Crystallized energy blocks of the "productive" variety can be characterized as follows: The client experiences an emotional response when he or she tries to enter the block (e.g., fear, disgust, nausea, pressure, etc.), and the client perceives a structures that can be entered such as bottomless holes, ponds, whirlpools, funnels, steps, doorways, passageways, caves, fires, cauldrons, tar pits, etc. Occasionally, you may find animated figures, dragons, magicians, and the like guarding or personifying the inner sanctum of the block.

What to Do With "Productive" Blocks

In dealing with the "productive" variety, it is essential that we enter the crystallized energy block, conquer all dragons, delve into the deepest recesses of the whirlpools, caves, etc., and overcome all fear or discomfort, until we are reasonably certain that we have arrived at the core of the block, feeling, memory, or experience. At that point, we may call on the Light for cleansing and healing. Usually, the various manifestations observed on the way to the core of the experience can then be dissolved easily.

Finding the Power Source of a Crystallized Energy Block

If a crystallized energy block does not yield completely, your next task is to find the power source that keeps it in place. This is important because without turning off the power supply it may either be impossible to dissolve the block -- or the block may easily reconstitute itself once the influx of higher-vibrational energy has diminished.

The power source may arise from a single spot in the energy body, or it may come from a complex network or "pipeline" system of blocks that all feed on each other and hook into several spots or chakras. In the latter case, we need to painstakingly dissect the system and uproot all its major branches before a lasting cleansing can be accomplished.[41]

You may approach the search for the power source from a number of angles. One possibility is to encase the crystallized energy block in golden-white light, in order to increase the contrast (again, "where there is more light, there is more shadow"). Then ask the client to look for a black power supply line branching off from the block and to trace this line to the place where it is anchored. The root of the black power supply line is most often a dark spot that can be found somewhere along the spine or in one of the major chakras. If the tracing of the power supply line takes you to a spot other than a major chakra or the spine, chances are that the block your client is perceiving first is just one of several blocks belonging to a more complex "pipeline" system. These systems may be rather involved, and activating one spot may send you to another and then to another and another.[42]

When this happens, it can get quite frustrating and taxing for all parties. However, tenacity and trust in the process

[41] This process is not unlike surgery on metastasized cancer. Often one does not know what one might find until the actual surgery takes place, and then one has to "dig" for as long as it takes. This is one of the reasons why flexibility in your schedule is desirable.

[42] Gary Craig, the founder of Emotional Freedom Techniques (EFT), calls this phenomenon "chasing the pain."

will pay off, in most cases. Here is a vignette to illustrate this point: One of my recent clients had a history of multiple severe traumas, including emotional and physical abuse, a near-drowning, a fire caused by lightning, and a near-fatal car accident. In the first session we had processed multiple incidents of emotional and physical abuse perpetrated by her father who, among other things, had forced her to eat glass. At our second session, I was aware of neither the drowning nor the fire. For quite some time we jumped from one crystallized energy block to another, without seeming to get anywhere. When my client reported seeing a red spot that looked like a flame, I took it for just another manifestation of a crystallized energy block. I encouraged her to go into the center of the flame. Suddenly she got in touch with a childhood trauma. As a nine-year-old, she had watched from her bedroom window as a huge burning tree -- which had been set ablaze by lightning -- fell onto her home. Paralyzed by terror, she was unable to scream for help; instead, she fainted, regaining consciousness as firefighters carried her from her home.

As we were working through the traumatic memories, she came to recognize a recurrent theme: In many of her traumatic experiences she had been unable to use her voice. She did not dare to speak up against her abusive, alcoholic father; she could not scream for help when she was under water gasping for air; and she could not scream when she and her family were in acute jeopardy even though she saw it coming. She dreamed about the car accident the night before it happened, yet in the moments before the accident, as she and her family approached the scene, she did not speak up -- even though she "knew" exactly what was about to happen. To add insult to injury, she blamed herself for having failed to prevent these events. Guilt, self-blame, and helplessness injure the throat chakra, and so it was no "accident" that she broke her second cervical vertebra in the car accident.

This client, a registered nurse, had taken heavy doses of pain medication[43] for many years. Medical doctors predicted lifelong debilitating pain and expected her to end up in a wheelchair. By the end of our first session, this client felt her spine shifting (without any manual manipulation), and after only two sessions, she has reported continued improvement in her range of motion and level of pain.

Although this story has many interesting aspects, I shared this case primarily to illustrate that the patient pursuit of systems of crystallized energy blocks, frustrating as it may be, can lead to important breakthroughs. Trust the process!

We have discussed the use of golden-white light as a "contrast medium." Another option is to enter the system at any point and trace the branch to its root. Your experience or intuition may assist you in locating this root. For instance, if the block shows up in the chest area, checking for a connection to the heart would be a good place to start. Often, as clients activate a peripheral block, I simultaneously feel a sensation in another area, most often a major chakra. Consequently, I may suggest that the client look in that area, rather than stay focused on a peripheral block. Thus, educated guesses and empathic perceptions may aid in locating the power source of a crystallized energy block.

Another technique is to ask the client's -- or your own -- inner guidance, or a being of Light, to indicate the place in the body where the power supply is located. Once the root has

---

[43] Pain medication or other pharmaceuticals are lower-vibrational in nature and may even be toxic. Prolonged exposure to toxins contributes to the formation of crystallized energy systems.

been identified, the client can enter the spot and decipher the information contained in it. After the power supply has been uprooted, or dried up, it is much easier to dissolve the original, crystallized energy block -- if the process has not already done so.

This and the previous chapter discussed the various manifestations of energetic blocks and what to do about them. The process can be summarized in four words: identify, investigate, transmute, and incorporate. *Identify* the block; *investigate* its nature and the information contained in it; *transmute* the energies contained in the block; and embrace, integrate, and *incorporate* the energies that were previously separated from the flow.

It is important to remember that you can never eradicate the energies contained in a block -- energy cannot be destroyed. All energy comes from Source and returns to Source; nothing is separate from Source. The process of transmutation -- the alchemy of healing -- cannot be dictated by your human mind. All we can do is allow the process to occur by revoking the barriers we have put in place.

As healer, you assist in the healing process, but you are not the source of healing. Trust the process! You are not doing this work alone. It is a collaboration between you and your client, your Higher Selves, your guides, and the beings of Light that collaborate with you. You are a coach, or pilot, whose role is to assist the client in navigating Inner Space. Develop a tolerance for uncertainty -- and a lot of patience. Balance what you know from your studies or from experience with your intuition. Avoid a cookie-cutter approach and stay tuned to your inner guidance and creative developments. Trust that with experience, you will get better at this -- and trust that there is always more to learn.

Chapter 14

Specific Techniques to Facilitate Healing

Once an energy block is breached, and its information is available to the client, there are many ways a healer may assist in the healing process. This chapter will present specific techniques that have proven useful.

Verbalization

Often it is helpful to put words to an experience. When you find the right words, or help your client to do so, they may deepen the experience, highlight its different aspects, foster cognitive integration and -- most importantly -- give the client a sense of being understood. When your empathic words hit the nail on the head, they dissolve barriers to awareness and thus bring about an inevitable energetic shift. This is, of course, the mechanism through which skillful talk therapy achieves its healing effects.

For an example, the client might remember a tonsillectomy at age three. You may describe the emotions this child is likely to have felt, such as fear, pain, abandonment, anger, powerlessness, confusion, etc. It helps to assist the "three-year-old" in sorting out his or her feelings with "adult" words, at once deepening the experience and making it more comprehensible and digestible.

In addition, verbalizations can help clients to get in touch with emotions that may not be readily accessible. A typical case is the experience of sexual abuse, which often brings with it feelings of shame, disgust, rage, hurt, mistrust, fear, confusion, violation, etc. Those are some of the feelings that are more easily identified. However, depending on the circumstances, it may also be necessary to acknowledge other aspects, such as sexual arousal or pleasure, or feeling special, powerful, desirable, etc. For a complete healing, we should strive to acknowledge *all* aspects of the client's experience, and a skillful verbalization can be very helpful in this regard.

Affirmations

Affirmations are positive, present tense statements that affirm something to be so.[44] Affirmations can have a powerful effect, instantaneously changing the flow of light throughout a client's body. The client's response to affirmations spoken while he or she is tuned in to Inner Space can be very interesting and educational. A typical situation that might call for the use of affirmations occurs with a client who harbors a deep sense of unworthiness. In response, we might ask the client to repeat the following affirmation three times: "I love and accept myself totally." There are two principle responses to such an affirmation: One possibility is that the client will be unable to speak these words with conviction, or even to speak them at all. In that case, we look for the place that holds the resistance or "talks back." The other possibility is that the affirmation

---

[44] "I AM strong and healthy" is one such example, as opposed to "I will not get sick" (which contains a negation) or "I will become stronger and healthier" (which refers to some point in the future). We capitalize I AM in reference to the I AM-Presence, another term for Higher Self or Totality. For other examples and details on the nature, function, and form of affirmations, we refer you to our publication *Affirmations and Thought Forms,* as well as Chapter 22 on Complementary Healing Techniques.

will cause an instantaneous shift, indicated by the noticeable influx of healing energies.

Another typical situation in which affirmations may be extremely useful is with a client who feels a deep sense of shame or guilt. Affirming aloud that "I release all guilt and I forgive, accept, and love myself completely" may give the healing process a significant boost.

When a client appears ambivalent or resistant, having him or her repeat a phrase such as "I wish to know what I need to know in order to heal" can lower the barriers to awareness. Other useful affirmations are: "I AM worthy of the Light," to balance a sense of unworthiness; "I AM healed and whole in the Light," to affirm ongoing healing; "I AM a powerful being of Light and I claim my power as co-creator," to redress a sense of disempowerment.

You can also make up your own affirmations, as the situation requires. There are no magic formulas. Allow your inspiration and creativity to create a phrase that is tailored to the needs of the client. Observing his or her response in Inner Space will tell you whether your suggestions are hitting the mark.

Imagery

There is no limit to the creative use of imagery in the healing process. Drawing on inner resources, the client will often develop his or her own imagery, which should be supported and incorporated into the healing process. The following paragraphs, however, deal with imagery suggested by the healer based on his or her intuition and inspiration. Here are three examples:

(1) If a past-life review has revealed repeated trauma of the same sort or with the same players, it may not be practical or necessary to address each scene individually. Instead, you may suggest a wholesale cleansing. Ask the client to "imagine a stack of slides depicting all the related scenes and a whirlwind of violet Light burning through them, cleansing all karmic entanglements throughout time and space."

(2) A client remembers and re-experiences a drowning experience when he was a young boy. He sees himself at the bottom of a swimming pool. You may suggest that the pool be filled with violet water and that he can release all fear, pain, feelings of asphyxiation, etc. into the violet water, merging with it instead of fighting it.

(3) A client feels terrified and abandoned during a traumatic event in her childhood. You may ask her to open to an awareness of the presence of her "guardian angel," her Higher Self, or another being of Light during that experience. Once she has a sense of a presence, ask her to merge with that being of Light as she goes through the traumatic event. This will most certainly change the energetic imprint of the experience.

All three examples have in common the fact that the suggested imagery is designed to work on an *energetic* level, not only a mental one. This is different from the use of imagery as a *psychological* tool, e.g., when you imagine being "Tarzan" in times of vulnerability or being "at a safe place" when you experience anxiety. Such mental imagery tends to be more of a palliative tool, whereas imagery designed to use healing energies becomes a powerful instrument of true healing.

Pyramids

Pyramids function like magnifying glasses for higher-vibrational energies. They act as portals to the higher planes. Often it is useful to introduce a pyramid of light into a scene from the past, the present, or even the future. For instance, when a client remembers a traumatic experience, we frequently suggest placing a pyramid filled with violet light over the entire scene. We encourage the client to visualize this light as it penetrates all the players, feelings, words, images, sounds, places, etc. that make up the experience. Once the entire "movie" has been played back within that higher-vibrational space and the transformation process appears complete, the golden-white light may be called upon to seal in the healing.

Calling in One's Higher Self

A unique application of imagery and/or affirmations is the suggestion to call the Higher Self into the heart through repeatedly affirming, "I AM that I AM." We have dubbed this ancient formula the "call letters of one's Higher Self" -- similar to letter codes used in ham radio or aeronautical communications. This formula works especially well if the client has a past life connection to meditations or invocations focusing on the Higher Self. In addition to -- or in lieu of -- this invocation, the client could visualize a bright diamond of golden-white light steadily intensifying and expanding in his or her heart. Then wait and see what happens. If the client does experience the conscious influx of Higher Self energy, this experience alone is bound to have a deep and transformative impact. It may be particularly helpful for those clients who need to release a sense of self that is limited, worthless, or powerless.

If the client is able to open to his or her Higher Self, just sit back and get out of the way. If you feel prompted by your inner guidance, encourage the client to engage in a dialogue with his or her Higher Self, for instance by asking, "Is there any thought, feeling or message your Totality might wish to share with you?" Any genuine "communication" from the Higher Self will have the quality of boundless, unconditional love, peace, and joy. Tapping into one's connection to Source through one's heart is a very profound experience that is inevitably transformative and healing.

Discourse

Usually, when the client is attuned to the heightened state of awareness we call Inner Space, we de-emphasize the normal human thinking processes. Generally, we do not want the mind to get in the way of the inner work. At times, however, it may be helpful to engage some of the client's more cognitive faculties, especially if there seems to be a need for deeper understanding.

For example, a mother may struggle with guilt feelings and a sense of having failed her children. At that point it may be opportune to share the thought that all parents feel guilty at times and that it is not the parents' job to make their children happy -- and vice versa. We might add that children and parents choose each other not for the comfort of the match but for the growth opportunities their relationship provides. There is always a long and intense karmic history between all parties and such history is usually quite mixed. Thus, it is not surprising that families are at once the source of the greatest joy and the greatest sorrow -- in fact, that is how it is designed to be!

It is not the purpose of such a discourse to convince your client of your philosophical views. Its purpose is to alleviate a client's suffering -- suffering that often appears unnecessary from a metaphysically inspired point of view. There is no hard and fast rule for when to engage in such extended discourse. Use your intuition and inner wisdom, as in all circumstances. If the discourse has hit its mark, it should open the door to an energetic shift that your client will be able to observe in Inner Space.

Invoking Guidance and Help from Beings of Light

At times it may be wiser to invoke inner guidance from a being of Light, rather than to engage in person-to-person discourse. Depending on the client's ability to perceive intuitively, calling on an Ascended Master, angel, Archangel, another being of Light (Jesus, Mother Mary, a saint or guru, etc.), or the person's Higher Self may prove most useful. The healer can then suggest questions to pose to the being of Light and ask for verbalization of the answers. This will come most easily through the "eyes"; the client will sense rather than hear a response. This could lead to a powerful three-way dialogue, provided that the "connection" is clear.

If you had asked your client beforehand whether he or she had the ability to channel, for instance, Archangel Michael or Mother Mary, most would have considered such a question ludicrous. In fact, that is exactly what happens with some clients while they are working in Inner Space.

A typical situation in which guidance from a being of Light could be most useful would be the case of someone who cannot forgive him- or herself (or others) for a certain action. Guidance regarding issues such as karma, (self-) judgment, unconditional Love, etc. may be more readily received if it is coming from a trusted being of Light rather than from another human being.

Working directly with a being of Light can help clients in several other ways.[45] (1) If a client is ambivalent about opening to an awareness to a traumatic experience, receiving help and guidance on the higher planes can provide the sense of support that tips the scale. (2) If a client has localized an area that appears too scary to penetrate, he or she may wish to call for reinforcement by a being of Light. Once your client senses a presence, suggest that he or she and the being of Light jointly enter the space of darkness or fear. (3) You can heal a situation or experience by blending the energies of a being of Light with the energies in need of healing. This is a variation on the theme of invoking healing colors.

Sound and Toning

Working with sound is just another way of working with energy. It can be used in many creative ways; and we encourage you to follow your intuition and to experiment in this domain. We will mention three typical applications we have found useful in our work.

(1) *Dissolution of energy blocks*: Most readers are probably familiar with the biblical story of the trumpets of

[45] See our publication *Angels and Other Beings of Light* for further details.

Jericho. Sound can indeed be used to break up fortifications and encrustations typically found around crystallized energy blocks. In my work I use Tibetan bells, a large crystal bowl, and my own voice. Other instruments, such as a tin whistle or cymbals, could also be used. The bells and bowl I use in my office create a continuous sound if you run a mallet or some other tool around the rim until the instrument vibrates consistently. This normally has a more profound effect than individual rings or strikes.

The sounds that I have been inspired to make with my voice range from disharmonious to harmonious, high to low pitch, moderate to loud, comforting to scary. I allow inspiration to take over and, at times, I am surprised by the sounds that do come out.

When using my voice to break up energy blocks I typically make a loud, sustained, high-pitched sound from the back of my throat that is hard to describe on paper. In any event, it would not get me a job at the opera! This sound is not intended to be harmonious or pleasant and often it is not -- but it is very effective. Before I use any kind of sound for the first time, I inform my clients about it in a few words. After that, I tell them each time, in advance, that I will be making a sound, so that they don't get startled. Frequently I use this sound in combination with a whirlwind of violet light directed at the observed blockage. Then I ask for feedback regarding the intervention.

In over 90 percent of the applications, sound has a profound effect on crystallized energy blocks. Even in those cases where there is little or no apparent effect, the realization that the block appears impervious to sound is valuable information, indicating that we still have more work to do to uncover the roots and power supply of the crystallized energy block.

(2) *Distinction between a past life scene and a mirage*: Sometimes you cannot be immediately certain whether a client's visual perceptions are a mirage produced by a crystallized energy block or the beginning of a past-life recall or some other significant imagery. I sometimes make a vocal sound directed right "into" the image, while I ask the client to observe what happens in response to the sound. There are two possible reactions that have clear implications: Either the image vanishes completely or transforms into something else, which means that we are dealing with a mirage; or the image remains unchanged or becomes even more perceptible. The latter outcome is likely to lead to a past-life recall or other imagery that will contain useful information.

(3) *Sound used for cleansing, healing, and integration*: A continuous and harmonious sound can be used in conjunction with healing colors as a tool to promote cleansing or healing. Some clients like the effect of sound toward the end of a session, because it can help with the process of harmonization and integration. Occasionally, I ask clients to come up with a sound that appears just right and encourage them to make that sound themselves.

Healing Touch

Touch is undoubtedly the oldest and most universally applied healing modality. In the context of Psychoenergetic Healing, we focus on the energetic aspects and neglect the physical aspects of healing touch. Placing your hands on or above an area that is in need of healing may be used to jump-start or support the healing process. Make sure that your touch has pure intentions, and that your client does not misperceive it as inappropriate. It is always advisable to ask for permission before you touch your client.[46] If in doubt, holding your hands above the body may be the better part of wisdom.

Tapping

Tapping on specific meridian points based on the protocols of Emotional Freedom Techniques (EFT), Thought Field Therapy (TFT) or similar methods can be a very useful tool when you are working in Inner Space.[47] Meridian-based tapping techniques are not customarily used in this manner, but they can be adjusted accordingly. Since clients keep their eyes closed when they work in Inner Space, the healer is normally the one who does the tapping. Always ask permission before you touch the client. It may be helpful for you to familiarize the client with the tapping procedure before he or she enters into Inner Space.

Watch the energetic effects of tapping as perceived in Inner Space. Tapping on certain acupoints may cause your client to perceive bright flashes of colors. Some reports suggest that a round or two of tapping may weaken crystallized energy blocks significantly. In that sense, tapping serves a similar function in the healer's arsenal to the focused application of sound.

---

[46] The question of touch is a taboo subject for members of certain healing professions. If you feel uncomfortable, or your client does, or you feel that it would be inadvisable for other reasons, by all means abstain from touch. Holding your hands above the client's body, or focusing your energies intentionally, are alternatives that may work just as well.

[47] We will discuss meridian-based techniques in Chapter 22.

In lieu of the self-assessment customarily provided by the client in EFT or TFT,[48] we have the advantage of directly perceiving the effects of the tapping on the "X-ray screen" in Inner Space. It is always a good idea to check carefully and then, if the client perceives even the slightest trace of a residual block, to follow up with the usual application of healing light.

Breathing

Breathing is an automatic and largely unconscious activity that deserves far more attention than it normally receives. Proper breathing is essential to the flow of oxygen and vital energies throughout the body. It is our observation that clients with physical or emotional imbalances tend to take shallow breaths from the chest while they lock the diaphragm and abdomen.

Observing a client's breathing patterns -- and particularly any noticeable changes therein -- can provide valuable clues to what is happening on an emotional and physiological level during the session. We will discuss four situations in which we would pay special attention to breathing:

(1) One of the best instant *relaxation* techniques we have found is to make a "soft belly" like a baby. Most people are trained to hold in the abdomen, a habit that is less than healthful. A soft belly is a natural and very effective antidote to anxiety and tension. Occasionally, we instruct clients to inhale and exhale forcefully into the abdomen as if they were

---

[48] In most meridian-based techniques, the client is asked to rate the severity of a problem on a scale of "0" (lowest) to "10" (highest). These numbers are known as "subjective units of distress" (SUDs).

blowing up a balloon. Such an exercise can help to stretch the muscles of the abdomen and diaphragm and thus to release tension and habitual holding patterns.

(2) Occasionally, clients may work themselves into a state of such upset that they keep sobbing heavily. Their breathing becomes very shallow and rapid, more like gasping. If that state continues for some time and the client seems to have difficulty soothing him/herself, we may instruct the client to make a conscious effort to shift the breathing pattern into deep abdominal breathing. This tends to have an instantaneous *soothing* effect.

(3) Conscious breathing can also be used to *deepen one's connection with the physical and emotional bodies.* Some of the people we encounter in our work have developed a typical defense pattern that we interpret as a split between the spiritual and mental bodies, on the one side, and the emotional and physical bodies, on the other. These may be clients who have been meditating for many years and who may have had significant psychic and spiritual experiences. Nevertheless, they may present with long-standing physical and/or emotional problems that have not responded to the higher- vibrational energies encountered on the higher planes.

When working in Inner Space, some clients may have easy access to colors and altered states of consciousness while their perceptions appear strangely unemotional, disconnected, and happening "out there," instead of within. In those instances, we might instruct the client to place his or her awareness into the abdomen, breathing the light "into the belly" instead of seeing it float somewhere around the eyes. For those clients who routinely disconnect or even dissociate, breathing into the abdomen is a most useful technique to deepen their connection to and awareness of their physical and emotional bodies.

(4) As part of our *induction into Inner Space* we routinely encourage clients to breath deeply "into the belly button." The purpose of this instruction is to (a) bring about instant relaxation and (b) to deepen the client's awareness of the physical and emotional bodies.

Chapter 15

Closure and Integration

Finally, you have come to the end of the healing session. Either all the work that needed to be done has been accomplished, or you have reached the limits of time or endurance. At this point, I often ask the client to check in with his or her inner guidance to see whether there is anything else that needs to be addressed, or whether we are done for the day.

When it is time to bring the work in Inner Space to a close, some sort of formula may be in order, just as at the beginning of the session. I normally say something like: "Let us wrap things up for today. What healing color or colors present themselves to seal in our work?" When the client perceives a healing color, ask him or her to "open to that Light and to allow it to permeate the entire body, touching every cell, molecule, atom, subatomic particle, and all the small spaces in between." I may also ask the light to touch all the other times and places we may have addressed in our work, such as past lives. We thank the Light and all Light beings for their help and presence and we ask for ongoing healing, transformation, guidance, and blessings at all times. We close by giving thanks. Then I sit back and allow the client to "come back" at his or her own pace.

By all means, do not feel compelled to follow this formula. However, some sort of closure is needed, and the areas that have been worked on ought to be filled with healing and sealing light. A formula has the advantage of punctuating the work in a predictable fashion while we invoke further healing and acknowledge the source of healing by giving thanks.

Upon the return from Inner Space, always ask the client how he or she is doing. Lightheadedness or slight disorientation are not uncommon and will normally pass within 15 minutes. If they are needed, offer some water, food, or grounding exercise. If a grounding exercise is indicated, I often ask my clients to visualize themselves as a tree with roots deeply planted into the earth, connected to the heart of the earth, and with the crown of the tree opening to the heavens. Then I have them see themselves as a balanced "bridge of Light between the heavens and the earth."

If, in the course of the session, you realized important biographic connections or made relevant observations, this is the time to share your insights with the client. Some explanation of the healing process and the underlying principles may also be necessary. Often, however, you may advise your client not to try to "figure things out with the human mind," but to let the mind rest and to trust the process. In general, be attuned to the client's needs and limitations at the end of an intense experience.

Advise your clients, particularly first-timers, that any number of responses can be experienced after a session, ranging from complete peace to an emotional roller coaster ride. Tell them to allow any and all responses and experiences, and to ask for ongoing help and healing, as the process does not end the moment the client walks out of your office. If it is appropriate, tell them that sometimes things may get more uncomfortable before they get better. Encourage them to call you between sessions if they need to, and assure them that "sticking with it" is worth the effort. Remind your clients that all healing is possible!

Chapter 16

Homework and Aftercare

Not every session ends with a homework assignment, but it can be a useful way to move things along between sessions. Typical homework suggestions may include journaling, meditation, prayer, affirmations, visualization[49] as well as the suggestion to observe one's dreams and moods, or to read certain books.

Taking the time between sessions to sit and meditate is a particularly important part of your client's transformation process, because it furthers the healing initiated in the session and makes a "statement to the universe" that the client is serious about his or her transformation, which, in turn, accelerates the process of growth and healing. The value of meditating cannot be overemphasized; it is as essential as practicing an instrument between music lessons.

If a session was characterized by a particularly intense release of emotional baggage, we sometimes suggest that the client take a shower and change into fresh clothing, so that the "old" energy can be cleansed even more thoroughly from the auric field. Purifying the home with incense or cleansing one's jewelry in sea salt for 24 hours may also be advisable under such conditions.[50]

---

[49] More information on these topics can be found in Chapter 22 on "Complementary Healing Techniques," as well as in many publications from other authors.

[50] Sea salt may not be suitable for opals and other soft stones. -- We will address the topic of psychic hygienc in greater depth in Chapter 20.

Last but not least, a healer may discuss certain lifestyle changes, dietary adjustments, elimination of certain foods or beverages, supplementation with vitamins or minerals, or the use of herbs or natural remedies. Of course, you should always stay within your area of expertise and avoid practicing medicine without a license. Because such topics go well beyond the scope of this book, we shall not discuss these matters in any detail.

Chapter 17

Specific Applications of Psychoenergetic Healing

Working with Children

On several occasions throughout this book we have mentioned special considerations that apply to working with children. Energetic healing efforts can be directed to children of any age, including *in utero* and even before conception. I am aware that such a statement sounds rather "over the top," if not outright crazy, but it is true. On the higher planes, a child is in contact with his or her future parents long before the time of conception. The soul of the child may actually have been involved in getting the parents together in the first place.[51] If one of the parents is psychically gifted, he or she can sense the nature of a child in waiting. Consulting a responsible and gifted psychic could also provide useful information. Whatever the nature, background, or needs of the future child may be, it can be helpful to invoke blessings and to request healing for the light body of the child, so that the possible effects of energetic scar tissue left behind from past embodiments may be mitigated in preparation for the anticipated incarnation.

---

[51] This could be the reason why Cupid is traditionally depicted in the form of a human infant with wings, aiming at adults with their bows and arrows and causing their targets of choice to fall in love with each other. We discuss this topic in greater detail in our publication *Angels and Other Beings of Light.*

Remember, all manifest creations originate on the higher planes.

If one of the parents or an energetic healer has the ability to work on the higher planes, there is no limit to the degree of communication and healing that can occur before, during, or after the pregnancy, regardless of the state of development on the physical plane. In principle, such work on the higher planes would not be any different from the healing of past lives or absentee healing. In any event, whether the parents have a detailed awareness of the child's energetic status or not, invoking blessings and healing for themselves, the child, and their relationship is always a good idea.[52]

As soon as a child is able to focus attention for a few minutes and to name colors, you can apply some basic Psychoenergetic Healing techniques. Use your creativity to adjust your techniques, imagery, and language to the developmental age of the child. For instance, I might ask the child to call on the violet friend, and have the violet guy get into a big fight with the black guy, so that they wrestle and get mixed up in each other. Or I may suggest that the violet guy tries to eat up the black guy like a birthday cake, until there is not even a little crumb of the black left.

Children tend to achieve easy access to Inner Space, often within seconds, and frequently they do not need to keep their eyes closed to remain in that heightened state of awareness. The natural psychic abilities of most children, and the fact that they are not confined by adult concepts of reality,

---

[52] In addition to working on the higher planes, there are many other ways one could work energetically with an infant or toddler, including Reiki, Polarity, Reflexology, acupressure, meridian tapping, and infant massage, to name a few.

makes working with children easier in some regards. On the other hand, they are prone to confabulation, restlessness, and shorter attention spans, and generally lack an awareness of more remote emotional events -- the flip side of living in the moment. This makes them poor historians and thus, they are often unable to identify the origin of an energetic block.

Depending on the developmental age, the child may or may not have the necessary discipline and tenacity to work through crystallized energy blocks or traumatic experiences. However, we have found that healing can usually occur even though the child may not understand the genesis of an energetic block, or the information contained within it. We can only hypothesize that there appears to be a "grace factor" at work.

In general, children are much more "fluid" than adults (i.e., a lot of energetic healing can occur in a brief period of time). The drawback to this fluidity is that the healing may not "stick" as well as it does in adults.[53] The energetic plasticity of children is one of the many reasons why working with the entire energetic environment, particularly with the mother and/or father, is very desirable.

If, for whatever reason, the child is unable or unwilling to do the energetic healing work, there is always the possibility of working with the child by proxy, i.e., by accessing Inner Space through the mother or father. This is a variation on the theme of absentee healing, which we will discuss at a later point.

---

[53] There is an obvious parallel to the physical domain: Children can get sick much more rapidly than adults -- and they can get well again just as easily.

With child clients, the healing of past-life issues may need some creative adjustments. For instance, an eight-year-old boy seemed to be overly fascinated by fighter airplanes and war stories. Although we had only circumstantial evidence to go by, the mother and I entertained the idea that he might have been an air force aviator who was killed in action in a recent lifetime. So, while working in Inner Space, I engaged the boy in a fantasy game and asked him to imagine that he was sitting in a fighter plane, and to tell me the story of what would happen next. Then we developed that theme and played through some "what if" scenarios along the lines of our hypothesis. Although our exercise did not provide a clear-cut confirmation, his preoccupation with fighter planes and war stories decreased significantly after this session.

Many children have memories of past incarnations or even of the time between incarnations. My godchild, for instance, a very bright and psychically gifted girl, occasionally spoke when she was five or six about her time in "baby land," a term she coined for the higher planes she inhabited before her recent incarnation. Others may say things like, "Mom, remember when I was a grown-up . . . ?" References of this kind are often ignored, misunderstood or even ridiculed, which is one of the reasons that children older than seven tend to loose touch with their earlier awareness of otherworldly realms.

The same is true for the phenomenon of "imaginary friends" or "imaginary playmates," which most psychologists regard as figments of a child's imagination. Little do these experts know that the higher planes are, indeed, populated by a wide range of beings, from the lowest to the highest. Some of these beings may become "guardian angels" or playmates to a child. Others, particularly those that belong to the lower astral planes, may take delight in scaring children -- which could be the source of many typical childhood fears and nightmares. Instead of telling the child categorically that there are no such things as ghosts and "things that go bump in the night," a parent or therapist should entertain the idea that the child may perceive something that is, indeed, quite real on another frequency. If the parent or therapist has a reasonable understanding of metaphysical principles and the basics of psychic hygiene,[54] he or she could truly help by changing the energetic force field in and around the child that attracts phenomena of the scary kind. In addition, the child could be appropriately educated regarding his or her own powers to change such experiences; for instance, he or she could be taught to call in higher-vibrational beings of Light and/or to put up light structures (such as a dome or pyramid of light) over the bedroom and home before going to bed.[55]

As we explained at the beginning of this book, we are living in a time of rapidly changing and accelerating frequencies. Children born today naturally carry a much higher frequency than those of us who have been incarnated for some time.[56] Thus, they have easier access to the higher planes in this time when the gap is closing and the veil is thinning. If we continue to treat these children according to paradigms that

---

[54] Chapter 20 will address the topics of psychic hygiene and the energetic cleansing of spaces.

[55] There are sound metaphysical reasons for the tradition of good-night prayers. In fact, a traditional Jewish prayer invokes the same set of Archangels to come to one's bedside as we invoke when setting up a higher-vibrational work space.

[56] The futurists Gordon-Michael Scallion and Cynthia Keyes present some interesting ideas on this subject in their audio-tapes on *Children of the Blue Ray* and *Children of the Rainbow,* published by Matrix Institute, P. O. Box 336, Chesterfield, NH 03443-0336; www.matrixinstitute.com; 800-628-7493.

simply do not apply anymore, at best we will be inefficient, and at worst we may cause serious harm. Those who are in positions of power regarding future generations need to wake up. The crystallized institutions of medicine, psychology, religion, and education, along with the mind-set of the past, will just not be appropriate to the needs of the children of today and tomorrow.

Addictions

At this point in the evolution of humankind, addictions can be found in one form or another in every human being. *Addictions*, as we define them, are habitual patterns of behaving, feeling, or thinking that do not serve the highest good of the individual. They are self-administered anesthetics designed to manipulate a person's inner states (moods, feelings, thoughts, perceptions, level of arousal, sense of self, etc.). Their function and effect is to avoid awareness or experience of certain inner states. They are motivated, in the final analysis, by fear.

There are innumerable "things" that can become the object of an addiction.
Among the obvious are alcohol and other mind-altering substances such as cocaine. (Substance abuse of this kind is not compatible with Psychoenergetic Healing. Only after a client has quit any substance abuse is there a chance for successful energetic healing work.) Then there are cigarettes, foods, caffeine, sugar, soda pop, etc., which are often lower-vibrational in nature and cause a physical and energetic imbalance in a person's body.

Among the behavioral addictions there are addictions to dieting, work, sex, pornography, thrills and dangers, jogging, gambling, TV/Internet, perpetual "busy-ness," etc. Less obvious are those addictions that are primarily internal experiences. Many of us are addicted to stress: We habitually create or expose ourselves to situations that cause stress in our lives. Although we may claim that we are victims of circumstance, in truth, we actively create or seek these circumstances (the popularity of TV programs such as "ER" is just one of the many examples we could cite). For many human beings, a period of time without stress, activity, or entertainment is truly a frightening experience.[57] Even when there are no obvious external stressors at work, we tend to create mental stress by habitually allowing worrisome thoughts to fill our minds. While most of us would claim that we desire "inner peace," the fact is that we often actively engage in any number of thoughts and activities that run counter to our stated desire.

Addictions can also manifest in the interpersonal domain. While this is a topic that easily warrants an entire chapter, suffice it to point to the various destructive interpersonal patterns which have been the topic of many a self-help book: Co-dependency, chronic enabling, relating to others from a vantage point of victim-consciousness, social-emotional exploitation and "leaching," the "helper's syndrome," persistent

---

[57] Recently we observed a group of adolescents who were visiting the local Buddhist Temple for the first time and were asked to spend seven minutes in silent meditation (sitting). After only five minutes, there was a noticeable increase of restlessness, noise, and activity among these high school students. Another example along similar lines is the response many people display to the experience of being without electricity for a day or two during a power outage: Many reported being most disturbed by the unavailability of TV, Internet, or video entertainment and there seems to be an increase of domestic violence under such conditions.

domination, Don Juanism, and many other abusive and destructive modes of relating to others.

What does this mean for the practice of Psychoenergetic Healing? We already said that active substance abuse is an impediment to this kind of work. All other addictions -- and there are some in each and every client -- are grist for the mill. If we understand that addictions are self-administered anesthetics designed to prevent an awareness or experience of certain inner states, the course of action is obvious: We need to find out what thoughts, feelings, and/or energetic configurations are motivating and driving the addictive patterns. In that sense, we view and deal with addictions in much the same way as we deal with any other energetic block that interferes with the free flow and experience of the client's energies.

So far we have worked with two clients who came to us for the explicit purpose of smoking cessation. Both had tried various methods, including hypnosis and acupuncture, and yet felt unable to kick the habit. Both had a history of trauma and loss: One client had lost his sister and brother-in-law in a car accident, the other lost her father to lung disease when she was nine years old. The male client almost drowned as a child; in addition, we discovered a memory of a past life in which he had died from smoke inhalation during a fire. The female client nearly suffocated at the age of four when her sister pressed a pillow over her face. This frightened her so intensely that she had an out-of-body experience. In both cases, the act of smoking was reassuring to them, as it gave them a heightened awareness of inhaling: "As long as I smoke I have proof that I can breathe." At the same time, smoking impairs the breathing process, thus serving as a reminder of the unresolved trauma.

The dual function of addictions -- and of symptoms in general -- is noteworthy: Often they are simultaneously an unconscious attempt to "heal" a trauma as well as a continuous reminder that there is an energetic scar that is in need of true healing.

Healing of Physical Symptoms

Healing on the physical level is not any more difficult or valuable than healing on any other level. However, those who are still skeptical and are looking for proof that energetic healing really works may be more impressed by the disappearance of physical symptoms. How is it possible that severe and persistent symptoms that have prompted repeated emergency visits to a hospital could be released in one session? How is it possible that long-standing symptoms of chronic illness[58] can disappear without so much as a physical touch? How can that pain from a sprained ankle or a surgical wound simply vanish?

There are no miracles, as we customarily understand that term. Miracles are the natural order of things. They come to us repeatedly and reliably, if we get out of the way and allow the perfect order of the Universe to manifest. What appears miraculous can be more easily understood if we remember two basic premises: "All of creation is vibration" and "all material manifestations originate on the subtle planes." In the context of physical healing, that means that the manifestation

[58] There is no such thing as chronic illness *per se*. The label "chronic" says *nothing* about the illness; all it really means is that, for whatever reason, the health care provider has not been able to treat it successfully; otherwise it would not be chronic.

of physical symptoms, as well as their disappearance, is an expression of energies that originate on the non-material planes. If we address the disharmony on the energetic level, all healing is possible.

The basic dictum of traditional Chinese medicine is, "If there is pain, there is no free flow; if there is free flow, there is no pain." This insight is as true today as it has been for millennia. Pain is not caused by an aspirin-deficiency. The most basic manifestation of the energy of constriction in the physical body is pain; in the emotional body it is fear. Pain and fear are two sides of the same coin. There is no pain without fear.[59]

How do you go about healing pain and other physical symptoms? You approach such energies in exactly the same way as you would any other energies that get in the way of a "free flow." In a nutshell, focus on the spot that holds the greatest intensity, open to an awareness of the information contained in those areas, ask for healing, receive, and trust.

The only variation on the information provided in other parts of this book pertains to "simple" physical healing, for example, of injured tissue around a surgical incision, or other symptoms of "uncomplicated" origin. In those cases, it is not always necessary to extract information from the area in distress before healing can commence. It often suffices to simply invoke a healing color and see whether it can mix easily with the disharmonious energies. Pink and green are particularly suitable for restoring health to physical tissue, but keep in

---

[59] The reverse is not necessarily true. Manifestation "trickles down" from the higher to the lower planes, the emotional being a plane of lesser density than the material.

mind that the colors needed may vary from case to case and moment to moment.

Healing of Past-Life Issues

We have all lived hundreds if not thousands of lifetimes. Each experience in a human body has affected us to some degree and has left its trace in our energy body. However, not all past incarnations are equally relevant. The lifetimes that do come up for review during the work in Inner Space are lifetimes that had a significant impact *and* pertain to the lessons on the agenda for the current incarnation. Thus, in all likelihood, we will encounter those past lives that left a significant amount of emotional scar tissue, and those that are related to the players and the script of the present lifetime.

Not surprisingly, the majority of sessions involving past-life recall deal with severe physical and/or emotional trauma. The kind of trauma reported from past lives often exceeds the worst any seasoned trauma specialist would ever encounter, for two reasons: In many of the lifetimes under review the events led to the demise of the protagonist; obviously, trauma with lethal consequences is not the domain of conventional psychotherapists. The second reason has to do with the fact that, generally speaking, past historic periods were often even more violent, dangerous, or cruel than today's "civilized" era. Dealing with trauma of such severity could be very hard on both the client and the healer were it not for the gift of healing, which can be so profound and rewarding.

The intensity of a client's experience varies with the nature of the story and his or her temperament and perceptual skills in Inner Space. Some clients have more of a vague sense, with more or less affect, while others truly "become" the protagonist of the lifetime in question and experience the story in full living color, including sounds, smells, and physical sensations.

I have never had such a "multimedia" experience myself, in contrast to Linda, who can recall any number of details from lives past. My sense of my own past lives is rather hazy. The way I *know* that such experiences really happened is by the intensity of emotions that I have experienced. At times I have been shaken so deeply by my recollections that I sobbed and heaved uncontrollably. Tapping into these veins of emotion has rivaled in intensity any other emotional experience that I have had in my life. In summary, a person's recall of a past life can range from vague to crystal clear, and from emotionally neutral to extremely intense. And these dimensions can be fairly independent from each other. Again, each person and situation is unique.

Having witnessed or experienced the intensity and detail of some past-life recollections, there is little doubt in my mind that past lives are "real." Thus, when I am asked whether I believe in past lives, I typically answer: "No, I don't *believe* in past lives. If it rains and you get wet, would you say you believe in rain? You *know* that it rains; it is not a matter of belief."

This is not to say that we believe that all recollections from a past life are true and should be taken at face value. As we will discuss later (under the heading "Is Inner Space 'real'?"), it is of little consequence to our work whether a particular event "really" happened as recalled or reconstructed. We are not concerned with historical accuracy. All that matters is whether our work results in an energetic shift toward healing.

It should be noted that we rarely approach a session with the preconceived idea that "Today, we are going to look at past lives." Unlike some hypnotists who purposefully perform past life regressions, we allow the process to unfold in a less directed fashion. This is one of the reasons that we generally do not speak of "regressions" and instead prefer the term "recall."

As we work in Inner Space, past-life recall may occur without any induction or prompting. Sometimes clients just start seeing past life images, occasionally even in a first session. In other cases, we stumble upon such information quite unexpectedly in the process of mining the riches of Inner Space. All of a sudden, you hit upon a vein of gold, and then you follow where it takes you. An experienced healer, just like an experienced prospector, would know where to look and would be attuned to hunches and promising signs, but it still remains an unpredictable and at times surprising adventure.

Most entry points to past lives can be found in crystallized energy blocks of the productive variety or, less often, in simple energy blocks. Occasionally, the healer may simply throw out a question and see what happens. When we ask for a number, for instance, in response to the question of when an energy block was put in place, we may get a number such as "0" or "100." Such an answer may be either simply bogus or an attempt to suggest that the story behind the block occurred before the current incarnation ("0") or a long time ago ("100"), also pointing to a time before the current incarnation. We may then say, "OK, it seems that this may be related to something that happened in a past life. Just ask your inner guidance to take you to a time and a place that may have put the black ball into your belly" (or whatever the case may be). The simple question of whether there may be a past life connection is often enough to open the doors to an awareness of a scene, which then slowly develops into a story.

How, then, do we go about healing the emotional scar tissue left from past lives? We use essentially the same techniques as for current life issues. First, we help the client to become aware of as much information as is available or useful. We may ask whether there are people in the image, whom the client seems to be among the persons in the scene, whether the protagonist is male or female, what his or her age is, and so on. If the scene opens with a sense of a traumatic event, which is often but not always the case, we may elicit a sufficiently detailed description of the traumatic scene and then request information about what led up to the event or what happened afterwards.

At some point, we may ask whether the client recognizes any of the players from the past life as someone he or she has encountered in the present life. In some cases, there may be no recognizable continuity between the past and the present; in other cases, the client may realize that one or more characters from the past have reappeared in the present. Recognizing the connection between the past and the present is often a profound and emotional realization that can open the doors to deeper understanding and healing.

If a scene is in need of healing, we invoke a pyramid of light filled with a healing energy such as the violet light. Then we ask the client to review the entire scene and bathe it in healing radiance until the emotional charge has been dissolved and all participants and details have been immersed in transformative light.[60]

If a scene appears too traumatic for the client to examine, we may ask for the assistance of a being of Light who could enter the scene with the client. The presence of such a being is often reassuring enough for a client to open to an awareness of the traumatic events.

In those rare instances when the "flashback" from a past life appears too intense and overwhelming, instructing the client to step back and to watch the scene like a video on a TV screen can be appropriate. In general, however, we steer the client *into* the scene, rather than away from it.

As with any kind of severe trauma that occurred in a current lifetime, we would watch for indications of dissociation from the experience and propose measures to reconnect with the full experience of the event. This can be done with confidence, as we can trust that the impact of any traumatic past life event -- regardless of its nature -- can be healed, normally within the same session.

Once the client has reviewed the significant events from a past life, we would look at the protagonist's light body, often at the time of his or her transition (death), or at the moment of the greatest trauma, and thoroughly check for areas that are in need of healing. In other words, we would scan the light body of the client (as it manifested in the past embodiment) for the presence of simple or crystallized energy blocks. Accessing the information contained in such blocks and healing them is typically easier when you are working on a light

---

[60] Depending on the nature of the experiences, a more extensive healing of the entire scene and all the players involved in the karmic drama may be indicated. Chapter 18 will discuss this topic in greater detail.

body from the past, rather than on the client's current light body.

Looking closely at the light body from the past can often reveal additional details that were not apparent in the initial review. It can also shed light on more internal events such as feelings of guilt, self-hatred, helplessness, loss, and so on. Furthermore, curses and vows[61] uttered in a time of intense rage or despair can also pose significant obstacles to the flow of healing light and may only become apparent by examining the light body thoroughly.

Once the light body from the past appears complete (i.e., no hazy, missing, or distorted body parts), radiant, and harmonious, we can then call in a column of light over the light body and suggest that the protagonist may step into the light for further healing and transformation on the higher planes. If the light body can ascend into the light with ease, we can be reasonably certain that a significant degree of healing has been accomplished. In the less likely event that the light body hesitates to step into the light or appears to be tethered to the earth like a balloon on a string, further exploration and healing is indicated.

Upon completion of the healing work on the light body of the past, you should return to the starting point in the client's current light body and clean up any residual imprint that may still be in effect. A wholesale cleansing with the violet

---

[61] Curses and vows are crystallized thought forms which deserve special attention in the healing process. If a curse (e.g., "May you all go to hell") or a vow (e.g., "I will never trust women again") was uttered by the person in question, it is important to explicitly revoke the curse or vow. In some rare cases we have found energetic traces of a curse *directed toward* the person in question. Under such circumstances, we recommend invoking the aid of Archangel Michael in conjunction with the violet flame.

light or some other healing radiance may suffice. If the starting point was a crystallized energy block, have the client ascertain that no residual traces of such blockage exist.

Rarely is there cause to work on the same past life a second time. Should the client feel the need to return to a past life that he or she has already explored, we can assume that an aspect escaped our attention the first time around. A healing is complete when the traumatic event from the past has lost its energetic charge and faded into the background, where it will be reintegrated into a person's Totality in a more harmonious fashion. Concurrently, any physical symptoms that were related to "bleed through" from that particular past life may also disappear.

Working with "Aspects of Self"

When we speak of past lives, there is still an implication of time progressing like a vector from the past into the present and from the present into the future. As we said earlier, this concept of time, while the only one that makes intuitive sense to our human mind, is not applicable on the higher planes. Instead, we suggested that you think of time as a sphere, with all points in time being equidistant from the center, our Higher Self. I sometimes use a Koosh ball, its countless rubber bands each representing a lifetime, to illustrate how all of our lifetimes occur simultaneously. If you find yourself struggling with the idea that there is no such thing as past, present, and future, and that reality is in truth timeless, you are in good company. The concept of time as it applies to the higher planes may be nearly incomprehensible to our human mind.

So why do we even bother to bring up a topic that seems esoteric, if not impossible to comprehend? There are several reasons: First, we claim that we can, indeed, heal traumatic events that occurred hundreds or even thousands of years ago. We do not only mean that we can change how we feel or think about those events -- we believe that we can actually change what happened! You may argue that you cannot change history. That is true when you assume that the past is the past -- water under the bridge, so to speak. But it is not so, if you allow for the possibility that you can enter any given place on the sphere of time, and that you can alter anything that happened -- since nothing ever truly ceased to exist. Again, there is wisdom in the bumper sticker slogan, "It is never too late to have a happy childhood."

Another reason we bring up this subject has to do with what we have called "aspects of Self." A few of our clients are very psychically gifted and have the ability to access several life stories in a single session. As we worked with these clients, we realized that the concept of past lives was too narrow to accommodate the fact that they were reporting several lives that appeared to be set in the same historic period (for instance, the first half of the last century). We either have to dismiss such reports as bogus, or we have to adjust the way we think about past lives. If all happens simultaneously, there is essentially no difference between lives that are set in the same historic period and lives that were centuries apart. They all would be considered aspects of Self.[62]

You will probably never discuss any of these finer points with the majority of your clients. Referring to the lives

---

[62] Other metaphysical writers have proposed the concept of "parallel universes" which may or may not be a useful idea in this context.

discovered in Inner Space as past lives suffices, for most practical purposes. However, there is another reason why the concept of "aspects of Self" has some significance. A person may have gained skills, understanding, or wisdom in a past life that could be brought to bear on the present life, or on the healing of another past life. For instance, one very psychically gifted client of mine had a past life as a male who was a masterful fencer. Before she became aware of this lifetime, she joined the fencing team of her university -- to her own puzzlement, as she is not really athletically inclined. Once we uncovered her past life as an excellent fencer, we asked this aspect of her to blend with her present self -- particularly when she was engaged in fencing. Lo and behold, her fencing skills improved dramatically!

Several of our clients have had lifetimes in which they developed great gifts as healers or reached great heights of spiritual understanding. These accomplishments from the past are not necessarily lost. We can integrate them into the present life -- or we may ask these aspects of Self to work in Inner Space with another aspect of Self from the past that could benefit from wisdom, guidance, or healing. For instance, one client had been a "philosopher" in one of her past lives. When we were working on some of her other past lives, we occasionally called him in and asked for his wisdom and understanding. This is a variation on the technique of requesting insight and guidance from a being of Light, only in this instance, the being would be an aspect of Self.

Chapter 18

Absentee Healing of Others and of Extended Situations

Absentee healing refers to any intentional healing directed toward another who is not in one's immediate proximity, and with whom there is no direct contact (e.g., over the phone). Given the fact that on the higher planes the limits of time and space do not apply, absentee healing is essentially not any different from any other intentional healing. In our work, we apply absentee healing primarily in three situations: when working with parents on their children, when healing past life scenarios, and when healing extended situations.

Parent-child Absentee Healing

Before we can legitimately engage in absentee healing with individuals, we should ascertain that doing so would be karmically proper and in agreement with the targeted person's Higher Self. Generally, when the person in question is an adult who is currently in a physical body, we may offer some healing on the higher planes but we could not do the work for that individual. When the person in question is a child, the situation is somewhat different. When we work with a parent on his or her child, we ask for the consent of the child's Higher Self and dedicate the intended healing work to the highest good of all. Due to the responsibility of a parent for his or her child's welfare, and due to the fact that children may not have the capacity yet to actively collaborate in their healing, we usually ascertain that absentee healing would be karmically proper.

The energetic bonds between parent and child are the strongest of any energetic ties that we can have with another person. This fact makes parent-child absentee healing particularly powerful and rewarding. Having said that, how would we go about the actual healing work? We would set up a higher-vibrational energy field, guide the parent into Inner Space, invoke a pyramid of light on the higher planes, and invite the child -- or, more precisely, a higher-vibrational representation of the child -- into the pyramid. Then we could simply ask the child to share the thoughts or feelings that are in need of healing. The information we are looking for could be communicated by means of body posture or through facial expressions, as thoughts transmitted when "looking the child in the eyes," or as thoughts that register in the parent's heart. Most clients need surprisingly little or no instruction in these methods of communicating on the higher planes; the majority seems to know intuitively what to look for.

Having listened to the child in this manner, the parent, in turn, would respond to or otherwise acknowledge what has been shared and, in collaboration with the healer, ultimately invoke a healing energy on behalf of the child. Then the parent would observe how the child reacts in response. Often the child relaxes, smiles, or even starts dancing with joy. On the other hand, an angry adolescent who feels guilty, ashamed, and unworthy may have a harder time allowing a healing light into his or her light body. We would then explore the blocks and discuss the issues, all on the higher planes. With patience and persistence an energetic shift can ultimately be achieved in most cases.

We could also scan a child's light body for indications of energetic blocks, just as we would scan the client's light body in Inner Space. Then we would take it from there, using the same techniques we would use if we were working with someone physically present in our office. Provided that the proxy is sufficiently adept in Inner Space, there is basically no difference between working with a "real" client and working on someone *in absentia*. Most of the techniques described in this book, including past life and physical healing, can also be used for absentee healing.

We have anecdotal evidence that strongly suggests that parent-child absentee healing is not only a theoretical option that makes good sense metaphysically, but also that it actually works. Having experienced the positive effects of such work, the parent learns to appreciate the intense energetic bond between parent and child -- a bond that is second to none among human beings. This provides an opportunity for the parent to understand more deeply the power of his or her thoughts and feelings about the child. And it opens up many more options for working with children and adolescents, countering the sense of helplessness and frustration that plague so many parents.

Past-life Absentee Healing

The second principal application of absentee healing is in the arena of past-life healing. Let us take the following example: A client recalls a past life in which he was a settler on the American frontier. One day, he and his family were attacked and killed by American Indians. The client recognizes that some of his family members from the past are also members of his current family. Therefore, it would be in the best interests of all first to heal the client's light body from the past and then to offer healing to the others, one by one, who were killed in the same event. This would be a case of past-life absentee healing applied to individuals.

The same idea can be extended to larger groups: In the case of someone who died in a battle or as part of an event involving a large number of casualties, such as a natural disaster, we could set up a pyramid of light over the entire scene and ask for the healing of all and everyone involved, including the soil on which the event happened. The client would observe in Inner Space how the healing is progressing and whether a certain geographic area or group of people may be in need of additional attention. This would be a case of past-life absentee healing applied to extended situations.

Absentee Healing of Extended Situations

Of course, it is equally legitimate to direct one's intentional healing to larger situations such as accidents, epidemics, genocide, warfare, earthquakes, wildfires, or floods. Absentee healing can also be applied to other, less dramatic situations: A client may live in a neighborhood or household where there is a lot of tension and negativity, or work in an environment which is less than harmonious -- the list of possible applications is inexhaustible. Do not underestimate the beneficial effects of such large-scale healing work!

One of our clients was a teacher in a special education setting for emotionally and behaviorally challenging middle school students. One evening she called in exasperation, ready to quit her job because "the kids were just impossible." Linda encouraged the client to apply what she had learned about working on the higher planes: setting up pyramids over her classroom and her school, calling in Archangel Michael, invoking the Violet Flame, etc. A week later she called and reported that there had been an immediate and perceptible shift in the behavior and atmosphere in her classroom. She continued to apply her metaphysical awareness in her work and quickly regained her sense of mastery and effectiveness as a teacher.

Invoking pyramids of light, asking for help from the higher planes and infusing healing frequencies into an event -- past, present, or future -- is never a wasted effort. It is always useful. Most human beings do not understand the power they carry in co-creating the world in which they live. Absentee healing is one of major ways we can put our power of co-creation to good use.

Chapter 19

Healing of Relationships

General Principles of Relationship Healing

Problems and disharmonies that may have developed in a relationship between two people are always caused by both parties. While we are often inclined to point the finger at the other person, the truth is it takes two to turn a relationship disharmonious. However, it only takes one person to heal disharmonies on the higher planes.

How can we heal relationships unilaterally? Again, we would go into Inner Space, set up a pyramid of light, and invoke the energetic presence of the other person inside the pyramid. Then we would exchange and share our thoughts and feelings, with as much honesty and intensity as may be needed. And, of course, we listen to the other person, in turn. Then we invoke a healing radiance, such as the violet or the blue of Archangel Michael, and fill the entire pyramid and all players within it with the light. We would observe whether the light can penetrate all parties completely and, if that is the case, we can be reasonably certain that a healing of the relationship has occurred. This simple "technique" may suffice for most cases.

If there are intense energetic bonds between two people, such as between a husband and wife at the brink of a divorce or between "victim" and "perpetrator" in an abuse situation, we may ask the client to visualize both parties stand ing face to face in the pyramid. Then we would ask to check for any energetic bonds or ties ("like rubber bands between the two of you"), their color and their location. For instance, the client may report, "there is a red cord between him and me at the belly button and another one, this one is more black, at the throat." If the observed connection is anything less than higher-vibrational in nature, we would proceed with an exploration of the "docking station" in the light body of the client, i.e., the place where the energetic cord has been anchored. Invariably, the "docking station" would be an energetic block in the client's light body, which we would penetrate and transform in the usual manner.

Once all anchoring points have been dissolved, we would ask for the help of Archangel Michael to sever all negative energetic and karmic ties between the two beings. The remaining ends should be "burned up like a fuse on a fire cracker." Throughout the process, we may check periodically until the client reports the absence of lower-vibrational energetic connections between the two parties. Note that this healing work can be done unilaterally and exclusively on the higher planes. Often there is no need or desire on the part of the client to follow up with any action on the earth plane, for instance, in a letter or some other form of communication, although that always remains an option.

Healing the Prenatal Mother-Child Relationship

The energetic interaction between a mother and a soul wishing to incarnate begins long before the process of conception. After conception, while the child is maturing *in utero*, an energetic barrier develops between mother and child. This barrier may be put in place by the mother as a manifestation of her fears and ambivalence and/or by the child, if the energies between mother and child are less than harmonious and the child desires a shield against the mother's energy field. As we have learned from the Ascended Masters, at this point in the development of humankind all unborn children grow up with such an energetic barrier in place. This is not the case for other mammals.

The Masters have suggested a powerful healing exercise that can be transformative for both the mother and the child regardless of their chronological age. Here is what we may say while working in Inner Space:

> "See yourself in your mother's womb as a tiny baby, with the umbilical cord connecting you and your mother. . . . Then notice a shield around the uterus, such as a dark or gray layer, or some other indication of a barrier separating the energies within the womb from the energies around it. . . . Then focus on the heart of the baby and connect it to an 'umbilical cord of light' that comes straight from Source, filling your heart and your entire body *in utero* with golden-white light. . . . See the light flowing through each chakra, lighting them up like a Christmas tree: glowing red at the tip of your spine, orange around the navel, yellow in the solar plexus area, green in the heart chakra, blue in the throat, indigo in the forehead/Third Eye, and violet and gold at the crown of the head. . . . Once you feel the radiant flow of light throughout your body, reach out and use this light to touch the energetic barrier around the uterus. . . . See how this barrier is dissolving. . . . Then see how the light is spreading beyond the womb throughout your mother's body, mak-

ing her radiant and filled with light. . . . Then let yourself be born and see yourself slowly maturing through all the stages of your life, while you keep intact the umbilical cord of light that connects your heart directly with Source."

This exercise tends to have a deeply healing and relaxing effect on both parties. If a mother wishes to offer this exercise to her child -- as yet unborn or born many years ago -- we adjust the healing exercise accordingly.

Healing the Child-Parent Relationship

A slightly different case from the one discussed under the heading of "parent-child absentee healing" is the reverse and more common scenario, when the client is working on healing the relationship with his or her parent(s). All of us have "issues" with our parents, and our clients are, of course, no exception. Thus, calling one's father or mother into the pyramid and working through relationship wounds and disharmonious feelings on the higher planes is a very useful and frequently employed technique.

As we have stated, the energetic ties between parent and child are the closest and most immediate connections between any two persons. Consequently, it is inevitable that an energetic shift in one party will affect the other -- for better or worse. Thus, working with *both* parties in the pyramid is particularly powerful. In some cases, the energetic interchange of the whole family will shift as one central relationship is being transformed. Of course, whether the parent accepts the offer of healing energies is up to him or her. In our experience, however, parents are often much more approachable on the higher planes than on the earth plane. Even if a parent has passed on, healing of the relationship is still possible.

Healing the Relationship with a Deceased Person

Many who feel they have some unfinished business with a deceased person are burdened by sorrow, guilt, regret, or other painful emotions. They feel that it is too late to speak their truth, apologize, or express love once someone has died. This unfortunate illusion has caused immeasurable suffering for many. The truth is that no one ever "dies" -- we only change form. Remember, all that has ever been continues to exist on the higher planes. Living is, indeed, forever. Consequently, there is really nothing that stands in the way of healing whatever unfinished business one may have with another, whether that person exists on the earth plane or only on the higher planes.

It can be deeply moving to observe the relief and healing that occur on both sides many years or decades after the passing of one of the parties in a relationship that was in need of healing. The good news is, it is never too late.

Chapter 20

The Issue of Psychic Hygiene

Just as a surgeon would not perform surgery without appropriate attention to the necessity for clinical hygiene, an energetic healer should not perform " psychic surgery" without attention to the issue of psychic hygiene. A surgeon needs to make sure that the operating room is clean, as well as his or her instruments and hands. Analogously, we will discuss how to cleanse a space, an object, and a person.

Before we deal with any specifics, though, let us address a few general points. The universe is composed of light of different frequencies, some of which are more beneficial than others. It is wise to be aware of this reality, particularly when you are psychically sensitive, in the process of opening, or performing healing work.

However, there is never a reason to fear lower-vibrational energies. Fear, itself a lower vibration, would make you more susceptible to such energies, due to the principle that "like attracts like." Imagine a dark cave that has not seen the light in eons. If an explorer were to discover such a cave and turn on a flashlight, the darkness would vanish instantaneously, while the flashlight would remain unaffected by the darkness. The light can transform the darkness -- but not vice versa.

When you find yourself in an energetic space that is less than pure, ask for a higher-vibrational light to come to you. For instance, the Violet Flame, the Christ Light, the light of Archangel Michael, or your own Totality would be appropriate choices, if you wish to be more specific. Instead of empathically taking in the disharmonious energies, radiate the healing light the way a light bulb radiates visible light.

If you keep yourself energetically harmonious, disharmonious energies will run off you like water off a duck's back. Operating on the principle of "like attracts like," you can only "catch" disharmonious energies if there is a corresponding "hook" in your energy field. This is one of the reasons why it is imperative for any healer working with energies to conscientiously clean up his or her own energy body.[63]

The various methods of energetic cleansing, and there are many, can be categorized into "physical" and "metaphysical" approaches. All have in common, however, one powerful ingredient: intent. Whatever you do, do it with intent. Whether you light a candle, strike a gong, or invoke pyramids of light, your intention behind any of those actions is of paramount importance.

How to Cleanse a Space

Among the *physical* methods used for cleansing purposes is the application of the four elements: fire, water, earth, and air. For instance, you could light a candle (the element of fire) and carry it through the room, intentionally bringing light into every corner. You could sprinkle "holy water" or water mixed with essential oils into a room, a method that is particularly useful to fill a space with "good" energy after a cleansing has been performed. You could place amethysts or other stones (the element of earth) in a room for the explicit purpose of

[63] We will discuss this topic in greater detail later in this chapter as well as in Chapters 24 & 25.

cleansing or maintaining a higher-vibrational energy field. Or you could cleanse a space through the diffusion of essential oils or the burning of incense, e.g., frankincense or myrrh (the element of air). In the Native American tradition the burning of sage is customarily used for the purpose of cleansing a space or an energy field (a process called "smudging") prior to the performance of a sacred ceremony. Cleansing rituals of this kind have been performed by many religious traditions in temples and churches, or around altars, since time immemorial. Note well that these are not merely empty rituals but sound, metaphysically informed practices.

Another powerful physical means of cleansing a space is the use of sea salt sprinkled liberally in a room, particularly into its corners and "dark areas." After a day or two, the sea salt should be swept up and discarded. Last but not least, sound could be used for cleansing purposes. For instance, you could make harmonious sounds with bells, singing bowls, cymbals, gongs, chimes, etc., while simultaneously focusing your thoughts on the intention of cleansing the room energetically. Again, bells, gongs, and chimes have long been used in various religious traditions -- and for very good reasons.

Among the *metaphysical* means of cleansing are some methods that we have already mentioned. You may invoke a dome of light or a pyramid of light, to be anchored over a space, a building, a neighborhood, and so on. Additionally -- or by itself -- you may ask for the help and presence of the Archangels and/or other beings of light. The invocation of the Violet Flame or its associated Ascended Master, St. Germain, is particularly useful for cleansing purposes. In addition, you may choose to call on the light of Archangel Michael, for similar purposes.

How to Cleanse an Object

When we wish to use *physical* means to cleanse an object, such as a blanket after a bad dream, we most often use the method of smudging, i.e., we waft the smoke of the burning sage around the object while we focus our intent on the energetic cleansing. Other methods mentioned above, such as the use of cleansing waters, could also be adopted for the cleansing of objects. Sea salt is a particularly useful medium for the cleansing of crystals, gemstones, jewelry, and other objects worn on a person's body for extended periods of time[64]. It is a good idea to cleanse any such objects periodically, particularly after you have experienced a significant energetic shift. All you need to do is put them into a container and cover them with sea salt for at least 24 hours; then discard the salt. If you intend to wear jewelry that belonged to someone else, it is crucial to cleanse such objects before you introduce them into your auric field.

Any stone or crystal that is used in healing work or placed in a room for cleansing purposes should itself be cleansed and recharged periodically. Gemstones, semiprecious stones, and crystals can also be cleansed through prolonged exposure to sunlight or through bathing them in running water such as an unpolluted creek.

All the *metaphysical* methods mentioned above for the cleansing of a space can be similarly applied to the cleansing of an object. In addition, you can place your hands around an object while channeling cleansing and healing energies such as the Violet Flame through your hands into the object.

---

[64] Some of the softer stones may not be suited to exposure to sea salt.

How to Cleanse a Person

There are many different *physical* methods of cleansing, not all of which can be discussed in this paragraph. The most common method is the application of the element of water. A few examples that come to mind are the practice of baptism, the ritual bathing in the Ganges, or the dipping of one's fingers in a bowl of holy water typically found at the entrance to any Catholic church. Each time a person takes a shower or a bath, the cleansing effects go beyond the physical body and extend to the subtle energy bodies. You could intensify the energetic benefits by "fortifying" your bath water with apple cider vinegar, sea salt, and/or essential oils.

Another simple method is to burn incense or sage while swiping it through a person's auric field, moving the smoke up and down the torso and the extremities, both front and back. Swiping one's hands through a person's aura with the intention of cleansing is another method used often by touch healers, e.g., practitioners of Therapeutic Touch.[65] Other healers use crystals, essential oils, or sound for cleansing purposes -- the list is virtually endless.

There are also many different *metaphysical* methods of cleansing a person, a great number of which have been discussed in this book. Since this is, after all, one of our central themes, we trust that we need not repeat the information presented in previous chapters.

---

[65] Therapeutic Touch is a consciously directed energy exchange during which the practitioner uses the hands as a focus for facilitating healing of the auric field. This method, developed by Dolores Krieger and Dora Kunz, has found wide acceptance among nurses and other healing practitioners.

Specific Applications in the Practice of Psychoenergetic Healing

In the general practice of Psychoenergetic Healing, we are primarily concerned with three areas of psychic hygiene: the office or healing room, the client, and the healer. Generally, it is essential to cleanse a healing space before and/or after a session, using one or more of the means discussed above. The client and/or healer also may wish to cleanse their auric fields at the beginning or the end of a session. This can be easily done with the help of incense, or by silently invoking the aid of the Violet Flame and Archangel Michael. If an extraordinary amount of lower-vibrational energy was released in a session, we sometimes suggest that the client shower or bathe at home, and put on a fresh set of clothes.

It is imperative for the healer to attend to his or her energy body before, during, and after each session. When a client is sharing a particularly traumatic experience, it is useful for the healer to consciously breathe violet or golden-white light. After each session, the healer should call on the help of the Violet Flame and Archangel Michael to restore balance to his or her energy body. Pacing, centering, and nurturing oneself before and after each session are also essential in this line of work. Good habits of psychic hygiene are as crucial for an energetic healer as hand washing is for a nurse or physician.

Chapter 21

Miscellaneous Topics

The Role of Teaching and Coaching

Teaching may take the form of impromptu lectures, metaphors, anecdotes, reminder phrases, case vignettes, reading recommendations, and the like. You may choose to share relevant experiences from your own path. Depending on your gifts, teaching may even come in the form of formal voice channeling of a being of Light, such as an Ascended Master.

Coaching refers more to the way you encourage your client to go through the process of healing and to endure the ups and downs that are inevitable for anyone who embarks on the path of growth. This is where the healer's wisdom and experience, gained from "walking the Shaman's path," become an invaluable source of guidance and reassurance for both parties.

The importance of teaching and coaching varies from client to client and session to session. Obviously, preadolescent children need not understand with their minds what you are doing, and why. Most do not benefit from lengthy explanations, which may even confuse and distract them. At the other end are metaphysically inclined adults who wish to deepen their comprehension of applied metaphysics, the nature of reality, karma, past lives, the healing process, etc. Adolescents and adults who primarily desire symptom relief fall somewhere between these two ends of the spectrum.

Since the premises of Psychoenergetic Healing are not commonly understood, and since the process can become quite intense, it is important that the healer provide helpful guidance and wisdom. However, he or she should avoid preaching or proselytizing. Respect and honor your clients' truth, as well as your own, and listen to your inner guidance in regard to the timing and content of your comments.

The Role of Intuition and Empathy

Empathy is a crucial ingredient in many forms of psychotherapy. In my opinion, it is probably the most important contribution to the healing process that a traditional therapist can make, and I deeply appreciate its value. In the domain of Psychoenergetic Healing, however, empathy has a slightly different meaning and function. In our work, it is not quite so essential to empathize with the emotions of the client, as the emotional surface is less relevant for healing than the energetic core. This is not to say that we would not honor and respect a client's emotions and feelings; of course we would. But there is a limit to the benefits of empathic listening and reflecting.

Let's assume a widow comes to you with issues of arrested and unproductive mourning. She already knows that she is upset and sad, maybe even angry, so giving her yet another opportunity to cry while empathizing with her feelings and letting her know that such feelings are understandable will only go so far. It may actually be counterproductive. We have all heard of clients who emote endlessly and who walk out of the therapist's office feeling worse than when they walked in.

As practitioners of Psychoenergetic Healing, we would soon move beyond the surface emotions and look at the energy body to find the places where the painful emotions are lodged. Once the underlying energies have been transformed, the client's emotional state will improve, often within a very brief period of time. Thus, the conventional wisdom that a conventional therapist is likely to offer the grieving widow, that "these things need time to heal," may not at all be true.

In Psychoenergetic Healing, the role of empathy pertains more to the energetic level. As you open yourself to an empathic awareness of the client's energy field, you will learn to perceive energy blocks, images, feelings, or other sensations in your own energy field that are a reflection of the client's energies.

Each healer's intuitive gifts are unique and will expand as he or she grows and heals. At this point, I am not (yet) good at picking up images; Linda, by contrast, has superb psychic gifts that enable her to "see," "feel," and "hear" many things in great detail. However, my seeming handicap has not really been a hindrance to doing this work successfully. Over the years I have developed the ability to feel the client's energetic blocks in my own body, often before he or she has become aware of them. I even feel those blocks when I work over the phone with clients who are 3,000 miles away, or when we work on the energy body from a past incarnation. Time and space, as we have stated before, present no obstacle on the higher planes.

In order to do this work well, one needs to open oneself to intuitive guidance, listening to the still, small "voice" within. I have found that the more I practice that kind of listening, the better I get at it -- and the same is true for anyone who desires to open to his or her intuitive gifts. Have patience, and trust that your intuitive skills will expand in your own unique and perfect way.

Indications and Contraindications of Psychoenergetic Healing

In this book, we have said more than once "all healing is possible." And we have claimed that Psychoenergetic Healing can be successfully applied to any number of mental, emotional, and physical problems. Conventional wisdom should probably caution you to doubt such claims; "if it sounds too good to be true, it probably is." To clarify, we are not claiming that all *will* be healed, only that all healing is *possible*.

Whether a treatment has the effect we desire from our human point of view depends on countless factors, many of which we will never be able to understand completely. We *cannot* know a soul's agenda, and we *cannot* know *all* the factors that enter into a certain manifestation on the material plane. All we can do is to serve the Highest Good to the best of our abilities, and then let things unfold as they may. "Not my will, but thy will be done."

If we understand that our claims are based on the paradigmatic insight that *all* is energy, they may not sound quite as outrageous as they would if they were evaluated from within the outdated paradigms of conventional thinking. Indeed, there are no *a priori* limits to the indications for Psychoenergetic Healing -- and there are no true contraindications.

However, there are a few factors that can cause significant obstacles. (1) Religious fundamentalism or some other form of strong ideological resistance to the premises of this work may get in the way of a productive therapeutic alliance. (2) Ongoing substance abuse accompanied by little desire to kick the habit may run counter to any efforts to transform a client's energetic patterns. (3) Clients who smoke cigarettes are typically much harder to work with, as their systems tend to be polluted with lower-vibrational toxins that feed crystallized energy blocks. (4) Clients with schizophrenia or other psychotic illness may be too confused or medicated to do productive work in Inner Space. (5) Anyone who is taking in a continuous diet of lower-vibrational energies will have a wider gap to bridge, and thus will face an uphill battle, when working with higher-vibrational energies. The lower-vibrational energies may stem from any number of sources, including junk food, unhealthy beverages, drugs, medications, cigarettes, poor lifestyle choices, "bad company," or a steady diet of mental and emotional pollution that is so easily accessible through today's media and Internet channels.

Last but not least, the old joke still applies: "How many psychiatrists does it take to change a light bulb? Just one, but the bulb must be willing!" If the client is unwilling to make the effort to change, there is little you can do but pray and let it go. As the saying goes, you can lead a horse to water, but you can't make him drink.

Dealing with Ambivalence, Doubt, and Resistance

Ambivalence is the natural state of the human mind. We tend to be of at least two minds about just about anything. It is important to acknowledge this fact, not to fight it. If we tried to suppress any of the mental opinions that argue within our minds we would only add to our tension and confusion. It is better to develop a tolerance for ambivalence than to impose a truce in an eternal tug-of-war that can never be completely resolved as long as the human mind operates on a plane of duality. "Peace of mind" is a rather relative term, if not a contradiction in terms. To find true peace, we need to let go of our mental preoccupations and instead find access to the wisdom of our hearts.

Given the inevitability of ambivalence, it is not surprising that we all are also ambivalent about changing and healing. We are perpetually torn between the forces of expansion and contraction. We wish to grow and we are afraid of change. And we find ourselves too often oscillating between the pain of the known and the fear of the unknown. That is just the way it is, and it is wisest to accept this fact. What you resist, persists. Do not judge your clients' ambivalence, as you will find the same within yourself. Encourage your client to accept ambivalence as a normal experience in the healing process.

Doubt is also an attitude that is not surprising, given the extraordinary nature of the experiences in Inner Space. Beginners, especially, sometimes wonder if they weren't just making things up. Over time, the explicit or lingering doubt is likely to disappear. It may be opportune to reassure clients that their perceptions are appropriate and similar to what others have experienced in Inner Space. In addition, addressing their questions, as well as teaching and coaching (see above), can help to dispel doubts regarding the validity of their experiences.

As any therapist knows, *resistance* comes in many forms and many disguises. As long as the client is willing to do the work in Inner Space, we deal with resistance in the same way as we deal with any other energy block. We ask the client to find the spot in the body that is most resistant to doing this work, and then w address it appropriately. In the final analysis, all resistance is rooted in fear. If we resist resistance, we only add to the energetic logjam; remember, what you resist, persists. Accept resistance, and you open the door to change.

If, however, a client is unwilling to do the work in Inner Space, you should try to understand the nature of the resistance as best as you can. Empathize with the client at the same time as you attempt to keep the option of the energetic work open. If all else fails, let go of this client and work through any emotions of your own that may have been stirred up by this "failure." Check within yourself for resistance or judgments that might have contributed to the course of events. Be compassionate with yourself, and remember that we can never fully know all the factors that enter into any given event. Recognize that all are teachers for one another and that whatever happens is in perfect order -- even if you cannot see it at the time.

Is Inner Space "real"?

Earlier, we defined the term "Inner Space" as having two meanings: Inner Space denotes a heightened state of awareness. It also refers summarily to the levels of reality that can only be perceived in such a heightened state of awareness. Thus, the term denotes a way of perceiving a reality as well as the reality itself.

When we ask whether Inner Space is "real," we do not question whether there is a reality beyond the five senses. It has certainly become obvious to the reader that we do, indeed, acknowledge many levels of reality beyond the gross-material plane. Without such an assumption, this entire book would be pointless. Thus, the question addressed in this chapter pertains solely to the *perceptions* in Inner Space, whether what is being perceived in Inner Space deserves to be called "real," or whether it is merely a figment of the imagination, like a hallucination or a dream.

One can only work comfortably in Inner Space if one allows for a wider notion of "reality" than that defined by our five senses. Clearly, what is happening in Inner Space is very real on a number of counts:

(1) There is a significant degree of order and "systematic logic" to the work, probably more so than in the process of traditional psychotherapy.

(2) There are themes and perceptions of surprising similarity across individuals. While many of the perceptions in Inner Space are quite bizarre and at first sight non-sensical, there is a "method to the madness." It *is* possible to extract a great degree of information from these perceptions, if you know what to look for.

(3) While working in Inner Space, many clients have intense experiences that appear very real to them. Certainly, there are clients who may doubt for a long time whether they are "just making this stuff up." Then, again, there are sessions where the intensity and/or clarity of the perceptions leave no room for doubt: For the client and the observer, such experiences are *real.*

(4) Frequently, there are tangible effects such as symptom cessation, immediate pain relief, improved wound healing, "miraculous" changes in relationships, and so on, which can be observed on the gross-material plane.

However, we do *not* claim that you can really find (to name a few) menacing little figures, bubbling cauldrons, or metallic triangles anywhere in a person's body. In that sense, Inner Space is akin to a virtual reality, like dreams, computer simulations, or Hollywood movies. Those aren't "real," either, but they can have very profound effects on the observer.

Even though we concede that much that is being observed in Inner Space does not fit the criteria for "reality" as defined by our five senses, we do not consider this to be a weakness. In fact, we will argue below that this question is irrelevant for the purpose of healing.

The "False Memory" Debate

When dealing with individuals who have a known or suspected history of abuse, especially sexual abuse, it is important to explain the notion of "reality" underlying our work. Clients may come in with a vague sense that there may have been (sexual) abuse in their past, either because of their own recollection or due to a suggestion by a previous therapist. The latter scenario has given rise to the "false memory" debate that has brought much acrimony and polarization into courtrooms, families, the media, and professional organizations. As we see it, both sides are equally misled, because both base their arguments on a notion of "reality" that is, in truth, an illusion.

Here are a few comments we would like to make in this context: One could argue on philosophical grounds that there is no "objective" experience; all experiences and perceptions are filtered and interpreted through the consciousness of the perceiver. Whether or not one agrees with such an epistemological position on philosophical grounds, when it comes to subjective, emotional, and personal experiences it can hardly be denied that each individual has a unique experience of any given event. For instance, if you ask siblings who grew up in the same household about their childhood and their parents, each one would tell you a vastly different story. Who would be right, who would be wrong? Each perspective is as valid and true as any other.

In the personal domain that concerns us as healers, it really *does not matter* whether or not an event actually happened. If the client feels or thinks that a certain event happened, that is all that counts. For the purpose of healing, it is irrelevant whether a client actually was abducted by aliens or sexually abused as a child, or whether those were imaginary events. If we find energetic disturbances in a client's energy body that contain thoughts, feelings, or images suggesting a certain experience, we deal with it on the level of those energies. It is not necessary to determine whether the event in question actually happened or whether it was an imagined event, a past-life memory, a story taken from a Stephen King novel, or even bleed-through from a parallel universe. It simply does not matter.

Once the client understands this fundamental position, the burden of fact-finding can be lifted from the process of healing. Nor does the healer try to assume the role of detective, which is one of the most awkward traps any traditional therapist could fall into.

Many therapists subscribe to the notion of "victim" and "perpetrator," and they insist that it is important to bring the "truth" to light for its own sake, regardless of the potential costs. In addition to the costs claimed by the proponents of the "false memory syndrome," there are other significant drawbacks to this popular position. We believe that to insist on the "reality" of the abuse, and to maintain that "acknowledging what really happened" is essential for emotional healing, is misguided and a disservice to the client. It hinges treatment success to external facts, not internal experiences. This shifts the "locus of control" from the client to an external event and thus disempowers the client.

The insistence on the importance of external events limits the possibility for healing. That is one of the reasons why many "victims" linger in therapy for a decade or longer, often without significant improvement, when true healing might be achieved in only a few sessions.

Therapists need to be mindful of the attributional frameworks they offer their clients. When therapists emphasize that "it was not your fault" and that "something bad happened to you that was beyond your control," the client may experience some relief from guilt and shame -- at the expense of perpetuating the sense of disempowerment and victimization that is one of the most damaging effects of any abuse experience.

When the guilt of the "victim" is alleviated by blaming the "perpetrator," we gain a very questionable advantage. In the process, we abandon the therapeutic stance of love and compassion for all in favor of the role of detective and judge.

From a metaphysical perspective, we are co-creators of our experiences, not victims. We are all equal players on a level playing field. No one has the authority to judge another. Any judgment is based on conceit and ignorance. "Judge not, lest ye be judged" is still the better part of wisdom.

The proponents of the "false memory syndrome" argue that elaborate false memories may have been induced through the suggestions of overeager and irresponsible therapists when, in fact, no such malicious manipulations may have ever occurred. Instead, it is at least as likely that the client tapped into a past life memory ("bleed through") that was then bent to fit into the framework of the current lifetime, due to a misunderstanding of the nature of "reality" on the side of both the client and the therapist.

One of my recent clients was an experienced psychotherapist who mentioned in our first session that she suspected a history of early childhood sexual abuse by her father. However, in her past rounds of therapy she had been unable to ascertain the veracity of this suspicion. I told her that there may or may not have been such an experience, and that we would look at this from the vantage point of Inner Space. Even if we found indications of sexual abuse, I would not consider it nearly as grave a finding as would most traditional therapists. I assured her that all could be healed, whatever we found. In our second session, she spontaneously tapped into a past life that was filled with severe loss, massive trauma, and abuse. Among the many events from that lifetime was a recollection of being raped and beaten at the age of twelve by a male character whom she identified as her father in her current life. At this point in the process, we do not know whether her suspicion of abuse was based on bleed-through from that particular past life or a repetition of the drama in the current life. The good news is that it does not really matter.

Kundalini Energy

Kundalini is an energy generally not well known or understood outside the realm of Eastern spiritual traditions. Since it is a most powerful energy, however, any energetic healer should have a basic understanding of its workings and manifestations.

Traditionally, kundalini energy has also been called "serpent fire" or "serpent power." In Inner Space it is perceived as a white light. The seat of the kundalini is in the first chakra. In traditional texts this energy has been described as a coiled snake resting at the base of the spinal column. Once the kundalini awakens, the "snake" uncoils and rises along the spine. The ancient symbol of healers, the caduceus, represents this energy flow in its depiction of two serpents spiraling up a central staff. Fully uncoiled, this energy can infuse the Third Eye chakra, and enlightenment may be experienced. "If therefore thine eye be single, thy whole body shall be full of light" (Mt 6:22).

There are three reasons why the awakened serpent power has long been associated with healing: First, it is a very potent energy that can be utilized for healing purposes. Second, an energetic healer who is working toward becoming an evermore-effective channel for healing energies will sooner or later experience the awakening of the kundalini energy within. Third, a client who has achieved a sufficient degree of energetic health may experience the awakening of this energy in the course of the healing process.

What are the signs that indicate such awakening? The manifestations of kundalini vary from person to person and situation to situation. In some, the awakening process is slow and gradual, in others rapid and dramatic. There may be a partial or full awakening, and in some cases the serpent "goes back to sleep" for long periods of time. Often there is a sensation of warmth, heat, fever, or "hot flashes." There may be physical pain, insomnia, or emotional discomfort. It may even feel like one's inner organs are being shaken up or rearranged.

Any energetic block that this energy encounters in its path up the spine will be highlighted, in keeping with the rule "where there is more light, there is more shadow." Thus, the powerful nature of kundalini should be respected; it is not advisable to force a premature awakening before a person's energy body is prepared to handle the "high voltage." There have been cases reported of rapid and premature arousal of the kundalini that caused a "spiritual emergency" -- and even the loss of the person's sanity. We have never encountered anything like that in the course of our work, and we do not believe that Psychoenergetic Healing would trigger such an emergency. However, it is wise to be aware of the various possible manifestations of the kundalini energy and to treat the awakening process with respect. If a client appears to experience an awakening of the kundalini energy, allow the process to unfold gently. Pay close attention to those areas in the person's energy body that still contain energetic blocks and transform them using the techniques outlined in this book. Such diligence should go a long way toward ensuring a safe and fairly gentle unfolding of this most powerful energy.

Chapter 22

Complementary Healing Techniques

In this chapter we will discuss a few healing techniques that are compatible with and complementary to Psychoenergetic Healing. We will start with the most important first.

Meditation

Meditation and prayer can both be considered means of communication with higher-vibrational energies. Communication includes the basic steps of sending and/or receiving. Human beings are constantly sending and receiving energies through their chakra systems and energy fields. When we pray or meditate, we add a crucial element to this continuous exchange -- the element of *intention.* We can consider meditation a way of receiving with intention, and prayer as a way of sending with intention.

Since ancient times, different ways of meditating have been advocated as means to bring about greater awareness, self-realization, and spiritual advancement. All techniques are designed to facilitate an opening to higher-vibrational energies through quieting the mind. Much has been said and written about various meditation techniques, which include breathing, sitting, walking, concentrating or emptying one's mind, repeating a mantra, etc. We will keep matters simple and straightforward. There is no need to get hung-up on the technicalities of the right or wrong way of meditating.

We encourage all of our clients to meditate between sessions; it is as crucial as practicing your instrument between music lessons. Which instrument you choose -- or which meditation technique you prefer -- is largely a matter of choice. We encourage our clients to experiment with the various traditions until they find an approach that works for them. While discipline and steadfastness are useful virtues on the path to spiritual growth, you should avoid rigidity and dogmatism about a specific method. Listening to inner guidance will help to keep your meditative practice alive and thriving.

Here are some basic pointers:

- Turn off all telephones, radios, etc., and arrange for a few moments of silence.
- Find a quiet space, preferably one that you have dedicated to your spiritual practice. Each time you meditate in your "sacred space," you reinforce its higher-vibrational force field. However, meditation can be done anywhere.
- Sit comfortably with your spine erect, but not rigid.
- Set up a higher-vibrational energy field, e.g., by invoking pyramids of light and beings of light into your space.
- Take a few deep breaths and then ease into slow, deep, and rhythmic breathing into the abdomen.
- Focus on your breathing and try to let go of all thoughts as best as you can. If you notice mental chatter or restless thoughts, gently put them into your breath and let them "flow out." You may wish to keep a pen and paper handy, to write down any pressing thoughts you wish to remember, so that you can release them from your mind.

• You may choose to silently repeat a mantra in your mind, for instance, "OM," or "I AM Peace – I AM Love - I AM Light," while you focus on your heart.
• Invite a healing energy into your body, particularly your heart. Recommended colors are violet, blue, green, or golden-white. Relax and let this light fill your body from head to toe.
• Release all negative thoughts or feelings that you might encounter into the light, for healing and transformation.
• Initially, sit for a minimum of ten minutes. You can gradually extend your practice as long as you wish.
• Commit yourself to meditating daily. Meditating in the morning rather than at night may be more beneficial, because it sets the tone for the day, and you are less likely to enter into a "sleepitation."
• Be patient; meditating will come more easily with practice.

How can meditation be useful for healing purposes? The general answer is that all meditation is by definition healing, as it intentionally opens the human energy field to an interchange with higher-vibrational energies that brings it into greater harmony and balance.

More specifically, you can use meditation for specific healing purposes. Imagine the following example: You are trying to sit quietly and still your mind. As your focus of attention turns within, you may notice that your mind keeps going back to an argument you had with your spouse and that your solar plexus region is upset, causing discomfort in your abdomen. You acknowledge your perception. Focusing on the area of discomfort, you try to penetrate the pain and all feelings and thoughts associated with it, becoming as aware as possible of all that you are experiencing within. Whatever it may be, accept this awareness without judgment. Then, open yourself and ask for a healing. Whether you feel an immediate relief or not, trust the process and allow it to unfold.

Prayer

Many studies have shown prayer to be a powerful means of healing that rightly deserves a place in a chapter on healing techniques.[66] Many of us pray in some form or other, and most of us had some instruction as to when, what, and how to pray. Although this book is not concerned with any particular religious tradition, we feel that some comments on popular concepts of prayer are in order.

When praying, many people adopt a position of submission, speaking as a servant or slave would to a king, begging for their master's favor. We believe that this attitude is fundamentally misguided. When we think of ourselves as weak and lowly, we will be exactly as we think. The power of thought is such that we become what we think of ourselves. An attitude of lowliness, self-abasement, and meekness does nothing to "please the gods." It weakens our energy field, as well as the power of our prayers, and thus is *not* a useful approach. We are co-creators, not supplicants. If our attitude is one of separation, seeing "God" in the Heavens as a remote entity ruling over the lowly creatures on Earth, we deny our true nature and instead experience "the fear of the Lord." An

[66] Larry Dossey, M.D. has written several books on the power of prayer; see the list of suggested readings in the Appendix.

attitude of separation and fear is lower-vibrational and *not* a good basis for prayer.

Another misunderstanding is the intention of manipulation, asking God for intervention on our behalf to ensure a certain outcome. This would be the case if we prayed to win a war (remember, both sides are praying!), to achieve a certain goal ("Please God, let me get that promotion"), or to beg for a certain outcome ("God, please help my grandmother to recover from cancer"). In other words, when we come from an attitude of manipulation, we want "God" to do our will, not vice versa. A wiser approach is an attitude of praying for the highest good of all to manifest. Since we can never truly know with our human minds what the highest good of all is, it is best to leave the outcome open and to surrender in trust to our Higher Selves.

From a human perspective, comfort is desirable, and so is perfect health. From the perspective of our Higher Selves, growth is the overriding concern. The growth that can be achieved through an illness can be so significant for all the people touched by the illness, that this illness is indeed in the highest interests of all. The person afflicted by the illness may learn important lessons about surrender, giving up control, asking for and accepting help, releasing self-hatred, or learning about humility, gratitude, and compassion. Those caring for the afflicted person may learn about service, unconditional love, patience, the impermanence of all forms, etc. Both parties are certain to learn important karmic lessons and to balance their karma with each other. So, instead of using "God" as a weapon in the fight against illness, it is wiser to pray for alignment with and surrender to the highest good of all. This will bring about growth, inner peace, and harmony, which are at the heart of true healing.

In summary, the power of prayer is related to our power as co-creators and the law of free will. When we come from a position of surrender to and alignment with the highest good of all, our prayers must be answered; it cannot be otherwise. "Ask and you shall receive" (Jn 16:24). *Asking* is an important ingredient, as the beings of light honor the law of free will and will not come unbidden. *Trusting* is another, most important component. "Whatever you ask in prayer, believe that you have received it, and it will be yours" (Mk 11:24). This quote points to the importance of trust, as well as to another significant aspect: Many prayers are spoken from a position of lack, asking for something that is lacking in the present and wanted for the future. Instead, *affirm abundance*, affirm that you already have what you need, and *express your gratitude* in prayer. Last but not least, trust that your prayers are equally effective as the prayers of anyone else. *Don't give your power away* by relying on intercessors. The higher planes are a level playing field. Remember that this is an "equal opportunity universe."

Besides the underlying attitudes we have addressed above, is there a right or a wrong way of praying? As we understand it, there is no reason to be obsessed with the right words or formulas to be used in prayer. Most important is the energy you put into your words, whether you speak them aloud or silently. A prayer spoken from your heart, energized with sincerity and feeling, carries greater weight than a long-winded formula spoken in absent-mindedness. What matters more than any specific words are your attention, intention, and underlying attitudes.

Affirmations

Affirmations are another powerful healing tool. Given our understanding that all of creation originates on the subtle planes, it only makes sense to use affirmations to consciously plant the seeds for the manifestation of healing. Affirmations help to transform thoughts we no longer wish to carry, and to reinforce thoughts that nurture our well-being. They are especially useful in transforming deeply ingrained patterns of thinking, feeling, and behaving.[67]

Through repetition, and with attention and intention, we create new thought forms that serve as the seeds of manifestation. Of course, our power of manifesting is greatest when we align ourselves with the highest good of all. Hence, all that has been said in this regard about prayer also applies to affirmations.

Here are a few simple guidelines on how to create and use affirmations:

- Always use positive statements.
- Always stay in the present tense. That is the only moment that matters. (Avoid statements such as, "I will not get into an accident." Rather, use a phrase such as "I AM safe and sound on the road.")
- Ask that what you affirm be for the highest good of all.
- Release all expectation of how the affirmation will manifest. Leave yourself open to all possibilities.

---

[67] Our book *Affirmations and Thought Forms* addresses this topic in greater detail.

• Remember: You always get what you need -- not necessarily what you want! Trust the wisdom of what comes to you, once you put the process in motion. Be patient; there may be layers to work through.
• Understand that you will not get rid of anything. All creation, once created, exists eternally. You can only transform the thoughts you wish to change by releasing them into the light.

The following are a few examples of affirmations we have found helpful:

• "I am whole and healed in the Light. I allow healing radiance to fill me continuously."
• "I let go of all preconceived ideas of who I am becoming."
• "I am in the flow of abundance from the Infinite Source. I trust this flow and accept its gifts freely."
• "I (re-) dedicate myself to serving the Light."
• "I release all negative thought forms related to (health, relationships, job, etc.) and affirm that all is in perfect order."
• "I surrender to the Love of the Infinite Source and allow it to be my guiding force."
• "I trust that all things and events that come to me are for the highest good."
• "I release all fears and realize that there is nothing to fear."
• "I release all judgment, honoring and accepting all for whom they are."
• "There is an abundance of time, energy and resources to accomplish all I have chosen to do."

• "I trust in the perfect order of all things. I allow this flow to carry me in grace and trust."
• "I am worthy of the Light and Love from Infinite Source, and I accept it into my being with an open heart."

The above examples are just that, examples. Feel free to use your own words in a style and manner that feels natural to you. Allow your inner guidance to come up with suggestions that suit your needs at any given time -- and allow for the possibility that they may change.

Visualization

Visualization can be considered an alternative method of affirmation. Much of what has been said about prayer and affirmations also applies to this tool of healing and manifestation. When we use visualization with intention while in a meditative state, we apply the same universal principles through a different "medium," or on another "channel."

Just as a picture may be worth a thousand words, so are visualizations at times more suited to the task than affirmations. Visualizations can go beyond a mental exercise if we infuse our imagery with higher-vibrational energies. Particularly for healing purposes, seeing yourself (or another person) surrounded and permeated by healing light is very effective. Among the visualizations we employ on a regular basis are pyramids of healing light, often stacked in layers, enclosing a person, building, country, or even the entire globe. This is a quick and immediate way to send healing light.

Some people are more visual by nature; others find it very difficult to use imagery and visualization. In any event, we encourage you to experiment with this tool. If you find yourself having some difficulty, trust that visualizing will become easier with practice.

Energy Psychology: An Emerging Field

We are currently witnessing the emergence of a new field that has been named "energy psychology." In 1998, the *Association for Comprehensive Energy Psychology* (ACEP) was founded as a professional organization to provide a home for a wide array of energy-based treatment methods. These include aura-based, chakra-based, and meridian-based techniques.[68] Because this discipline is still in its early stages of development, it is constantly changing and shifting, and it is too early to tell which methods will ultimately prevail. At this point, meridian-based methods appear to enjoy particular popularity.

Over the past few years, there has been a proliferation of new psychotherapeutic techniques among the meridian-based methods, some of which we have already mentioned in earlier parts of this book. In my own work, I have successfully used *Thought Field Therapy* (TFT), developed by Roger Callahan, and the *Emotional Freedom Techniques* (EFT), developed by Gary Craig, either as a stand-alone technique or in conjunction with working in Inner Space. Other popular methods include the *Tapas Acupressure Technique* (TAT), developed by Elisabeth (Tapas) Fleming; the *Negative Affect Eras-*

---

[68] A brief synopsis of the various traditions influencing the field of "energy psychology" can be found in the Appendix.

ing Method (NAEM) developed by Fred Gallo; and *Be Set Free Fast* (BSFF), developed by Larry Nims.[69] New names and acronyms emerge frequently; therefore, we encourage you to do your own research, if you wish to keep abreast of the more recent developments.

In our experience, some of the theoretical premises and techniques developed in the domain of "energy psychology" are compatible with our own work. We do not claim that Psychoenergetic Healing is the final answer for all clients and all practitioners. We feel that there is room for many different approaches, and we are grateful for the emergence of "energy psychology," as it signifies that the overdue shift toward an energetic paradigm is finally, albeit slowly, taking hold in the world of psychology.

Energetic Touch Healing Techniques

There are numerous energetic touch healing techniques practiced in the healing arts. They range from the more physical (e.g., Reflexology, Shiatsu, Polarity) to the more non-physical (e.g., Reiki, Therapeutic Touch). Any of these healing techniques is useful, and we encourage appropriate training if you feel drawn to it. Linda and I have been trained in Reiki (II) and have received an Earth-energy attunement. In addition, I have been trained in massage, Reflexology, and Polarity balancing, and I have studied acupressure on my own. I frequently use my "proprietary mix" of acupressure, Polarity, and Reflexology, most often on a client's feet. I may choose to do some

[69] Web site addresses and/or other references can be found in the Appendix.

"foot work" while I am talking with my client before we start with the "light work" in Inner Space. It helps to balance the body's energy flow and tends to relax a client profoundly. Occasionally, the energetic blocks found in the body may lead directly to work in Inner Space.

There is ample room for experimenting with various energetic touch healing techniques and how they may complement the Psychoenergetic Healing work. Again, we are open to a variety of methods and would never discourage a mix-and-match approach to healing.

Nutritional Adjustments and Supplementation, Homeopathy, and Vibrational Remedies

Nutritional Adjustments and Supplementation

Many clients who present with emotional, mental, or spiritual imbalances also suffer from physical imbalances -- and vice versa. Thus, a comprehensive approach to healing would ideally attend to all four "bodies," including the physical. Very often an evaluation of a client's nutritional and metabolic status may be indicated. For example, a client may present with various symptoms of anxiety, insomnia, hyperactivity, etc. There may be an underlying metabolic imbalance that contributes to an overactive sympathetic nervous system and an inability to relax. In such cases, trying to affect a positive change on the emotional level while neglecting the physical imbalances can be an uphill battle -- if not entirely futile. A hair mineral analysis, for instance, can provide useful information on a client's metabolism and the potential need for the addition or elimination of certain supplements. If the area of your expertise -- or the scope of your license, if applicable --

does not extend to the physical realm, you should consider making a referral to an appropriate practitioner.

Homeopathy

Homeopathy is a complex system of healing that is very compatible with any energy-based approach. A number of our clients are taking homeopathic remedies that do not have the same detrimental effects on energy-based healing as do many pharmaceuticals. Finding the right homeopathic "constitutional remedy" can actually enhance and facilitate our work significantly. Thus, a professional relationship with a trustworthy homeopathic practitioner is highly desirable.

Vibrational Remedies

This category refers to a wide range of remedies that are designed to affect the healing process through their energetic properties. To name a few, essential oils as used in aromatherapy, flower essences, and gem elixirs belong in this category. In our own work, we occasionally recommend specific essential oils or Dr. Bach's Flower Essences. Since the basic premises of these remedies are highly compatible with our own approach, we find that a complementary use of vibrational remedies may be very beneficial.

PART III

Becoming a Psychoenergetic Healer

Chapter 23

Training in Psychoenergetic Healing

Just as studying a few books on surgery would not make you a qualified surgeon, there is more to becoming a Psychoenergetic Healer than reading this book. Part III of this book will discuss the process of becoming a Psychoenergetic Healer, starting with an outline of the formal training. The following chapter will address the risks and benefits of becoming a healer, and the last chapter covers some general comments on the processes of healing and growth that apply to everyone, client and healer alike.

Training in Psychoenergetic Healing

We founded the Institute of Psychoenergetic Healing and wrote this book because we wish to share our experience and to help others to develop their gifts as healers. Thus, teaching and training are very much part of our agenda, and we invite all who feel called to learn more to contact us.[70]

---

[70] Our postal address is Institute of Psychoenergetic Healing, P.O. Box 516, Chagrin Falls, OH 44022, USA. Our e-mail address is *expansion@u-r-light.com*; our web site is *www.u-r-light.com.*

Entry Requirements

Formal Requirements
While a background in the healing arts (e.g., counseling or mental health) can be useful, we have set no formal requirements for acceptance into training for Psychoenergetic Healers. You do not need to have a college degree or any other formal entry qualification. This is not to say that everybody has what it takes to become a Psychoenergetic Healer, or that the training is anything but rigorous, as you will see below.

Personal Requirements
More important than any diploma or formal course of study are personal attributes and characteristics of the person who wishes to become a healer. Below we will discuss desirable personal qualities and the crucial question of motivation.

Qualities: Here are a few desirable -- even indispensable -- qualities and characteristics we would wish to find in a healer-in-training (this list is neither exhaustive nor in order of importance):

- Scrupulous honesty toward self and others, and the courage to embrace one's shadow;
- An openness toward change and transformation on all levels;
- Intellectual flexibility and agility, and a capacity to entertain abstract thoughts and concepts;
- The ability to communicate well;
- The ability to connect empathically with others;
- A high degree of interpersonal and intrapersonal maturity;

- Integrity of character;
- Sensitivity regarding the feelings and needs of oneself and others;
- A caring, sincere, and compassionate heart.

Motivation

A fair amount of soul-searching should go into exploring the motivation behind one's desire to become a healer. In the New Age vernacular, the catchphrase "intent is everything" has become very popular -- and there is some truth to that. By "motivation," we mean the conscious and unconscious intent that fuels our thoughts, actions, and choices. Here are some of the questions we need to ask ourselves repeatedly: Do I wish to be a healer because it feels good to make a difference in other people's lives? Do I like the feeling of self-importance that comes from being privy to another's innermost secrets? Do I satisfy my own needs for closeness and intimacy by connecting with the client from the safety of being the "expert"? Do I enjoy the acclaim or admiration that comes with performing what seem to be "miracles"? Do I wish to heal my own issues through working on another person's pain? Do I wish to become rich, famous, or loved through doing the work?

We cannot tell you what the "right" answer to those questions should be. If you answered "no" to most or all of them, you may be less than truthful with yourself. Human beings are messy, and we all carry higher and lower aspects within ourselves. By addressing the question of motivation scrupulously, we can learn a lot about ourselves, and we may avert harm from our clients and, just as importantly, from ourselves. We shall discuss this topic in greater depth in Chapter 24, "Risks and Benefits of Becoming an Energetic Healer."

Training Components

The training can be broken down into didactic and experiential components, which we will elaborate on below. For further details of the training (format, duration, costs, and location), please contact us and/or visit our web site for updates.

Didactic Components

We will be offering introductory and advanced *seminars* to teach and demonstrate the theory and practice of Psychoenergetic Healing and related topics in the area of applied metaphysics.

Furthermore, *reading* assignments and recommendations will provide a theoretical foundation and give all participants a common frame of reference. However, the amount of required reading will be limited, as there is little written information at this point that is absolutely essential. Of course, many fine metaphysical books have been written that may be relevant although not directly related to Psychoenergetic Healing, and we encourage our students to explore the areas they are most interested in as they see fit.

We also plan on producing audio- and/or videotapes based on seminars, live demonstrations taped during trainings, and recorded sessions with actual clients.[71]

Experiential Components

As part of our seminars, there will be guided group *meditations,* so that all participants can experience the flow of ener-

[71] Please visit our web site *www.u-r-light.com* for available training materials.

gies within. In addition, your personal meditation practice is an essential element of your becoming a healer.

The second experiential component is the *observation* of Psychoenergetic Healing performed live or on tape, either by a teacher or a healer-in-training. Following each demonstration, there will be a time for sharing and a discussion of the "technical" aspects of the healing work.

The third experiential component consists of personal healing work or *self-healing*. In the next chapter, we will explain some of the issues that will undoubtedly rise to the surface in the course of your development as a healer. "Walking the shaman's path," as the phrase goes, requires that you learn to heal your own wounds first. By doing so, you acquire the qualifications, tools, and experience that will then allow you to assist others on their own paths toward self-healing.

More advanced healers-in-training who are practicing Psychoenergetic Healing with their own clients will receive *supervision* or consultation. Depending on individual needs and circumstances, there will be either a formal, ongoing arrangement to provide training through supervision, or consultations as needed, regarding a specific client or challenge.

Chapter 24

Risks and Benefits of Becoming an Energetic Healer

Let us assume that you are considering becoming a spiritual healer, a shaman, or a Psychoenergetic Healer. First, we could ask whether this is a matter of choice. Can you choose to become an energetic healer the way you would choose to go into law or auto mechanics? Or is it something you simply must do?

Of all the choices we might make in our lives, the decision to become an energetic healer is most similar to the decision to have a baby. As with becoming a mother, "walking the shaman's path" is stringent and arduous. It will transform you to the core of your being. Nor do the parallels to motherhood end here. Becoming a healer affords you the opportunity to experience the greatest joy, as well as the greatest pain and fear. It is not a hobby but a 24-hour-a-day job, requiring great dedication and discipline.

The practice of energetic healing assumes the presence of higher-vibrational energies, or Light, that can be used for healing purposes. An energetic healer is someone who has learned to connect with *and* channel these energies to the person, plant, or animal in need.[72] Energetic healers may differ in the ways they access higher-vibrational or healing energies. They may use rituals, prayer or invocations, trances or dances, symbols or visualizations -- whatever works within the belief

---

[72] Someone who uses prayer for healing may indirectly invoke healing energies by requesting intercession, but the one who is praying does not, in most cases, channel those energies through him- or herself.

system and cultural context of the healer and the one receiving healing. All energetic healers have in common, however, that they use themselves as the channel or entry point for higher-vibrational energies. They become vehicles or conduits of healing light.

What determines the level of vibration used in the healing process is not so much a particular path of access as the intentions of the healer, and his or her ability to become a clear and harmonious channel. When it comes to working with healing energies, a loving heart, and purity of spirit and intention, are far more important than specific invocations, procedures, or rituals.

In essence, an energetic healer is a *channel,* using his or her own energy field as a vehicle and tool for the healing work. The healing powers of an energetic healer are related to the level of energy that he or she has learned to access. In order for a healer to be a conduit for higher-vibrational energies, his or her physical, emotional, mental, and spiritual bodies have to be adjusted to those higher levels of energy. To use a crude metaphor, most ordinary people run on a voltage of 110 volts, some operate at 240, a few can process 1000 volts in their systems, and great masters can touch a high-voltage power line with impunity. As the Light is beneficent, it will only flow to the degree that one's system can handle it safely.

The energetic force field of the healer interacts with, and is affected by, the energies to which he or she is opening. When a healer opens to higher "voltages," all of his or her thoughts, feelings, and karmic patterns -- positive or negative -- become *amplified*. This is a most crucial point.

As we have stated before, "all of creation originates on the subtle planes." We co-create our world through the thoughts, emotions, and intentions that we carry. Due to the amplification process explained above, any disharmonious thoughts or feelings in the healer's energy field -- and we all carry those to some degree -- have the potential of manifesting more strongly and more rapidly.

What does this mean practically? Here are a few examples. Many shamans become physically or mentally ill as an expression of the disharmonious energies present in their force fields. In fact, in traditional cultures the healing crises shamans typically endured were considered the hallmark and initiation of true shamans. Closer to home, we may carry the fear of losing our license, the approval of our professional peers, or even our livelihood. Whatever our greatest fears are, they will tend to manifest with greater immediacy as a result of the "higher voltage" that is charging the energetic healer's force field.

Similarly, if a healer carries the slightest trace of judgment against a client, the client will surely sense this intuitively and may choose to judge the healer in return. If a healer feels sexually attracted to a client, that, too, can be felt energetically. If a healer is motivated by greed or fear of lack (a lower-vibrational energy), the flow of abundance will stop. If he or she is motivated by ego needs, such as the need for self-aggrandizement or adoration, a "sucker punch" from the universe may be right around the corner. Thus, it is imperative to be aware of one's motivation, and to keep that motivation as "clean" as possible.[73]

---

[73] Computer programmers have long used the phrase, "garbage in -- garbage out." In our context the formula for manifestation could be summarized as "garbage in + higher voltage = more garbage out, faster!"

While there is no safe and easy way of "walking the razor's edge," there are certain guidelines that can help along the way.

(1) *Vigilance and discipline*. "Know thyself." Become aware of what you are thinking, feeling, or speaking, either aloud or in your "self-talk." *Notice* when you indulge in judgment of yourself or others, when you entertain thoughts of unworthiness or lack, or when your thoughts or actions are motivated by fear. Vigilance and discipline are of the greatest importance at all times. This makes being an energetic healer literally a 24-hour occupation.

(2) *Asking for help*. Once you have noticed disharmonious thoughts or feelings don't try to suppress them ("what you resist, persists"). Instead, acknowledge them from the viewpoint of an observer, and ask for help! Ask the Light, your Totality, or the beings of Light to whom you feel most connected to transform and transmute those thoughts or feelings every time you encounter them -- and then, let them go and trust!

(3) *Affirmations and prayer*. You may choose to use positive affirmations to change your thought forms and thinking habits. Or you may pray for help and healing of your negativity.

(4) *Forgiving and loving yourself*. Whenever you encounter negativity within, acknowledge it, forgive yourself for it, and focus on learning to love yourself without judgment. If we can love everything about ourselves, we are well on the way to ultimate transformation.

(5) *Self-healing*. "Physician, heal thyself!" This ancient call to self-healing is crucial in the case of energetic healers. You may ask, "How do I progress on my inner journey toward self-healing? How do I know which way to turn?"

The answer is simple: Go where you want to go the least! If you want to advance, there is only one way to go: penetrate your resistance; encounter your greatest fears; look at what you hate to see the most.

Walking the shaman's path will inevitably lead to encounters with your inner demons. And there are no dragons more fierce and terrifying than the ones we harbor within ourselves. Through all times and all cultures, the myths of heroism and initiation have told the same story, albeit in different words and metaphors. It is the tale of going into the darkness, encountering terrifying demons, overcoming one's fears, and achieving mastery and self worth in the process. Some will feel that they are not up to the task, and that is okay, too. Those, however, who are determined to slay the dragon will gain strength, courage, wisdom, and life. This may prove significantly more demanding -- and rewarding -- than going to medical or graduate school.

We have established that the shaman's path is stringent and demanding. So why would anyone choose to walk that path? The final destination of the healer's journey is total transformation, self-knowledge, and self-realization. In other words, you do it for yourself (i.e., your Self). If, along the way, you happen to help a few clients toward their own self-healing and self-realization, that is fine. But they don't need you; they don't need "fixing," as they are in perfect order as they are. If you wish to serve God/Spirit/the Light, that is fine, too. But God doesn't need you, either. If you feel it is a calling, so be it. Realize, however, that it is a calling of yourself by your Self.

The only true motivation for walking the shaman's path is your soul's desire for complete transformation while you are in human form. This is the greatest adventure of all, the most demanding and rewarding job you could ever choose. It is like giving birth to yourself -- including labor pains, messes, and all. Your progress on the path is the training that allows you to help another do the same for him- or herself, provided that is your mutual agreement. And by healing yourself, you ultimately contribute to the healing of all. So -- what is your choice?

Chapter 25

The Process of Transformation and Change

As we stated early in this book, we live in a time of rapid change on all levels. Nothing is as it was nor as it will be. No human being is exempt from the need to transform *radically* (Latin for "down to the roots"). For the sake of simplicity, let us assume that there are two ways one may choose to respond: embracing change and actively pursuing it (i.e., the path of expansion); or resisting change and trying to stem the tide (i.e., the path of contraction). Each choice has consequences. We will now look at these options one at a time.

The Path of Resistance and Contraction

In this time of increased pressures toward change many (if not most) human beings, are choosing the path of resistance and contraction. Many will not feel worthy or strong enough to do the work necessary for inner growth; many are simply too confused and frightened; and some have explicitly chosen to align themselves with the forces of negativity.

All over the world human beings, out of confusion and fear, are trying to find refuge in fundamentalism, dogmatism, and self-righteousness. Many feel that others who may belong to a different tribe, race, nation, or creed have wronged them, and they cannot see an alternative to seeking revenge for perceived injustices. Many feel threatened by any difference they perceive, insisting that their own worldview, customs, creeds, and prejudices must prevail. Fear and narrow-mindedness thus fuel the many wars that are fought on this planet on any given day, whether in an armed conflict between nations, a gang war in a neighborhood, a war of words among political opponents, or a war among members of a church, community, or family.

When watching the news or reading a newspaper one may easily become convinced that the currents of negativity are growing stronger and stronger, threatening to drown out the last bit of Light on the planet. But that is not the case. While there is plenty of negativity to be observed, we are also witnessing opposite trends. For instance, there is an unprecedented rise in interest in all matters spiritual. Fifteen years ago, books with titles such as *Saved by the Light* or *Celestine Prophecy* would have never made it onto the best-seller lists. In the grand scheme of things, all is ultimately in balance. What we do see, however, is an increasingly sharper contrast between the energies of expansion and the energies of contraction.

While we all have witnessed enough of the manifestations of the force of contraction, there is reason to believe that we will be seeing even more such in the times to come. Why is this so?

The Dynamics of Change: Individual Choice and the Larger Picture

At this point, let us revisit a topic we addressed in the opening chapters of this book: the rapidly increasing influx of higher-vibrational energies into this corner of the universe. The Earth's energy field can be thought of as an *open system*, a system that is trying to maintain a balance within certain parameters but is subject to outside influences. Natural ecosystems have comparable characteristics. To use an example, nature tries to balance the population density of certain species in a given bioregion, but outside influences such as acid rain from sources hundreds of miles away may upset the balance. When there is enough pressure toward change, a system will destabilize, go through a period of rapid fluctuation, and ultimately reach a new level of balance. This is what is currently happening to the Earth's energy system. It is the nature of any system to resist change beyond a certain comfortable range until a change of the system's parameters becomes inevitable. We can then understand in terms of system dynamics why we are going through a time of heightened tension between the forces of expansion and contraction, leading to great fluctuations in the planet's energy field.

Of course, humanity is not just a passive recipient of the higher-vibrational energies infusing our planet. We actively interact with and attract these forces and co-create the process as it unfolds. Let us recall two of the basic premises spelled out in earlier chapters: (1) All is connected to everything, and there is no real separation between that which is "us" and that which is "not us." (2) The human energy field operates like a powerful antenna, simultaneously receiving and transmitting energies at all times. If we consider the implications of these assumptions, it is only logical to assume that we do, indeed, affect the energies presently flowing into the Earth's energy field.

Can we avert the transition of planet Earth into higher levels of vibration? No. We can resist it, but we cannot avert it. The more we resist it, the greater will be the calamities and the rougher will be the ride, but we cannot stem the tide. The process of transition and change slated for this part of creation was set in motion a long time ago. It is a crucible we co-created for the awakening of human consciousness from its deep state of forgetfulness. It has to be and it will be.

Now, where is my *free will* in all this, you may ask. Before we incarnated in human form we all had access to an awareness of the impending changes scheduled for this time on planet Earth. We all *chose* to be part of this! And there were many, many souls clamoring for a spot on the front lines, so to speak, as reflected in the unprecedented numbers of people inhabiting the Earth at this time.

Why did so many souls choose to come into a body at a time when there is a potential threat to the survival of many? As stated before, the path to soul growth -- what we called the curriculum in the school of life -- is determined by a being's Higher Self. The Higher Self is primarily interested in growth rather than comfort. One of the two principal avenues toward soul growth involves the balancing of karmic debts -- which are the consequences of past choices. Many souls have chosen to balance their karmic debts at this time through suffering or even disembodiment. Other are reaping the rewards of many lifetimes spent in service to the Light by having the opportunity to serve once again during a period of radical transformation.

The second principal avenue toward soul growth is the pursuit of growth itself. Since the current times are characterized by a quickening of vibrations and accelerated change, there now is significantly more soul growth possible in a much shorter period of time. The learning that may have taken several incarnations during other periods may now be accomplished in only one lifetime. In other words, we are like surfers taking advantage of a huge tidal wave for a swift and exciting ride into greater growth and expansion. If we cannot stem the tide, wouldn't it make sense if we tried to enjoy the ride and get as far ahead as we can?

Our prediction of a period of increasingly sharp contrast between the forces of expansion and contraction and of a time of turmoil on many levels may also be understood in another way, by use of a metaphor: Human beings need food, water, and air to breath so that we can metabolize the fuel we need to feed our physical bodies. In addition, we need subtle energies to feed our subtle energy bodies. "Man does not live by bread alone" (Deut 8:3). Just as we are used to a certain diet for our physical body, we are used to certain frequencies that are most compatible with our subtle energy bodies. When there is a major change in the kinds of foods available, either we adjust our body to the new source of sustenance or we will starve to death. This change is currently happening on the subtle energy levels, affecting all our bodies: We either adjust on a deep subatomic level and beyond, learning to digest thc new kinds of energies available, or we will ultimately "run out of air to breathe." This can be a very frightening experience for those who are unable or unwilling to convert to the new "fuel" that, at some point, will be the only fuel available.

We have said that human beings are not only receivers but also transmitters of energies. While we do not generate energies in the ultimate sense -- all energy stems from Source -- we do have the power to transform energies to a specific level of frequency. So, in a sense, we can generate some of the old "fuel" to keep us going for a while. And this is exactly what is happening. Many will choose to stoke the fires of hatred, anger, greed, confusion, and fear because it "energizes" them. With the lower-vibrational "air" getting thinner and thinner, they feel drawn to generate thoughts and feelings that would keep them supplied with the fuel they are used to.[74]

We can now understand why those who choose the path of resistance and contraction are ultimately an "endangered species." Many will assist the planetary transformation through transitioning, abandoning their physical vehicles like cars that have run out of gas on the side of the road. They may choose to find themselves in the path of natural or man-made disasters; they may simply give up and commit suicide in one form or another; or they may die from a multitude of illnesses, all of which can be traced back to an increased level of conflict and imbalance in their energetic bodies. Whatever the path of the individual, such choices need to be honored with compassion, rather than judged.

Those who choose the path of expansion, by contrast, affect the larger picture in a different manner. The more Light we carry, the more we can radiate these frequencies across the Earth plane. Thus, beings of Light who have opened themselves to these higher-vibrational frequencies become conduits or vessels for the Light, facilitating the influx of ever-increasing currents of Light. And indeed, the Earth is populated by thousands, if not millions, of light-bearers who have agreed to facilitate the transition process by functioning as entry points for these energies. As the "ground crew," these light-workers are an integral and pivotal part in the transition process, easing the birth pains of the New Age through their spreading of the Light. At this point, there are many more than "a thousand points of Light" actively at work, and ever more are awakening each day.

---

[74] If you have any doubt about the dynamics at play, think of the rush of lower-vibrational energy that is generated by riots, looting, or battle.

In summary, we all have to decide whether to align with the frequencies of contraction and resist change, or to open to the energies of expansion and welcome change. Each individual's free-will choice, of course, has consequences. We are by no means helpless victims of uncontrollable forces imposed upon us. Instead, all of us who chose to be born at this pivotal time are given the privilege and responsibility of being co-creators in an evolutionary process of unprecedented proportions.

The Path of Growth and Expansion

Stages of Change

As we stated before, change is the natural order of the universe. There is nothing that remains unchanged or static forever. The universe is constantly changing, evolving, and expanding. Even the ground under our feet, seemingly solid, is shifting at all times. The crust of the Earth, the tectonic plates, is drifting, rising and falling, suspended on a core of molten matter that is whirling around with astonishing swiftness. The more strongly the tectonic plates "hang on" to each other -- the greater the resistance to movement -- the stronger will be the earthquake that results when the resistance succumbs to the pressures of change. This principle also applies to the human experience.

While each person's journey is different, radical change tends to follow a sequence of steps or stages:

(1) *Destruction*: This stage is often the most frightening, and can be compared to an earthquake. Your world as you

know it is falling apart; you may lose a loved one, your livelihood, home, health, family, etc. You may go through a divorce and in the process lose all your friends, your social identity and societal status, your source of income, and so on. Or you may have inner or outer experiences that shatter your view of the world. No matter what this may be, a common characteristic of these events is that you would not readily choose to experience them.

(2) *Deconstruction*: After the first major "earthquake" is over, the dust begins to settle and you sort through the rubble, selecting those bits and pieces that may still be of use in the future. In this stage, "aftershocks" may still occur frequently, contributing to the deconstruction process.

(3) *Reconstruction*: Recovering from the shock waves, you try to reassemble your world in a new way. As the phoenix arose reborn from the ashes, new growth occurs after the fields are burnt. This can be a very fruitful time of accelerated growth and expansion.

(4) *Integration*: The last stage is a time to settle in and integrate your experiences on a new level. You are given an opportunity to recover and consolidate your growth, gaining strength until the cycle may start anew.

We have outlined these stages of radical change so that, should you find yourself in its midst, you will have at least some idea of where you are and where you are headed. We hope that, sketchy as it is, this road map may also assist you in guiding your clients through an experience of radical change.

The Dark Night of the Soul

A very common experience on the path to growth and expansion is a period of extended and intensified struggle, confusion, despair, loneliness, and doubt. It is so common an experience that it has earned a fitting label, "the dark night of the soul." Jesus endured it, St. John of the Cross described it, and many, if not all, fellow travelers on the path have been visited by this spell of darkness. When you find yourself in a time of great challenge and struggle, when everything seems to go wrong, when your spirit feels defeated and you feel alone and confused, remember that it is always darkest before the dawn. This is the time of your greatest tests. If you wish to reach the peak of light, you must traverse the valley of the shadow. Know that, while you have to go through this alone, you are not alone in the experience.

And you are not alone in yet another sense. There are many beings of Light standing by, ready to help you the moment you ask. When you feel most separate from Source, or when you feel like hiding from the Light, pause and ask for help, and help *must* come. It cannot be otherwise. Trust.

Travel Tips for the Road

The following list is far from exhaustive, but it is a good place to start. Remember, the truth is simple.

- Be patient with yourself. There are layers upon layers, peaks and valleys, and times when everything seems to be at a standstill.

- Have compassion for yourself; don't judge yourself harshly. It wouldn't be a worthwhile challenge if you scored 100 percent on each test.
- You don't need to be "perfect" to deserve love. Personal and spiritual growth is uneven and oftentimes messy. If you have stumbled on your path, pick yourself up and move on. Forgive yourself!
- "You gain some, you lose some." As you are changing, your circle of friends is likely to change. You may experience periods of loneliness or isolation. This is a normal experience for all who change rapidly. Remember that our relationships are reflections of ourselves. As we change from within, these changes will be reflected in our relationships around us. Do not expect your partner to change and grow at the same pace or in the same direction. However, you may expect your growth to create changes in your partnership.
- Honor each individual's path. Don't preach or proselytize (a beginner's mistake), but share freely when asked.
- If you find yourself judging others harshly, look within and heal what you cannot accept in yourself. Remember, others are merely your mirrors.
- Be honest with yourself and others.
- Be vigilant and diligent in your pursuit of truth.
- No matter how far you have come, and no matter how wondrous the gifts may be that you have developed, be watchful for the traps of the ego. You are neither better nor more worthy than any other being. Beware of conceit. Practice humility. All are equal in the Light.

- Look closely at what is in front of you. Usually, you find the greatest teachers and most important lessons right under your nose.
- Don't think that you have arrived. There is no final destination. There are only temporary rest stops along the way (if you are lucky). The path is the goal.
- Keep humor alive -- it can save your sanity!
- Approach life with open hands; don't try to cling to anything or anyone.
- Go with the flow. Accept what is, don't try to resist; infuse all your experiences with healing Light.
- Practice love, compassion, and trust in all matters.

The Fruits of Transformation

If walking the path of growth and expansion amounts to so much hard work, you may rightfully ask, "Is it worth it?" You will have to decide for yourself. It often feels inevitable, as if refusing to grow is just not an option. The Higher Self is a tough taskmaster, and when life keeps hurting you badly enough, eventually you just start doing the work. Most stumble onto this path kicking and screaming. Few volunteer with grace. But this, too, is your choice.

While there cannot be an end to the growth process -- there is no final destination -- there are many fruits along the way. You may find, among other things, greater wisdom and inner peace; more love and compassion in your heart; increased awareness; psychic and spiritual gifts; a deeper sense of oneness with your Light and all there is; and a greater appreciation of the ceaseless wonders of life. You may let go of many of your fears and give up many of your judgments. And you may come to feel that you are doing your life's work, that you have found what you came here for in the first place: to grow, to expand, and to learn in the school of life.

Appendix A

Energy Psychology: A Synopsis

The following overview lists 12 traditions -- as well as the names of their founders or major representatives -- that have contributed to the emerging field of Energy Psychology.[75]

Ancient Traditions

(1) Chakra/Prana Lineage (India)
Yoga, Pranic Healing, Pranic Psychotherapy
Barbara Brennan, Rosalyn Bruyere, Caroline Myss, Choa Kok Sui

(2) Meridian/Acupoints/Qi Lineage (China)
Acupuncture, Acupressure, Shiatsu, Qi Gong, [Feng Shui]

(3) Aura Lineage

(4) Shamanism

(5) Religious Lineage
Prayer, Exorcism/"casting out of spirits"

---

[75] This overview is based in part on "The Energy Psychology Desktop Companion" by David Grudermeyer, Ph.D., co-founder of the Association for Comprehensive Energy Psychology (ACEP). He can be contacted at Willingness Works; phone: 800-915-3606; e-mail: drgrudemeyer@willingness.com.

Recent Developments

(6) Nursing Lineage

Therapeutic Touch (aura), Healing Touch (aura and chakra)

Dolores Krieger and Dora Kunz (TT)

(7) Physical Therapy Lineage

Kinesiology

(8) Chiropractic Lineage

Applied Kinesiology, Touch for Health, Educational Kinesiology, Neuro-Emotional Technique, Total Body Modification

George Goodheart (AK), John Thie (TFH), Dennison and Teplitz (Edu-K), Gym and Walker (NET), Victor Frank (TBM)

(9) Touch Healing Lineage

Healing Touch, Therapeutic Touch, Reiki, Radiance Technique, Polarity, etc.

(10) Psychology Lineage

Callahan Techniques/Thought Field Therapy, Behavioral Kinesiology, Emotional Freedom Techniques, etc.

Roger Callahan (TFT), John Diamond, Gary Craig (EFT), Greg Nicosia, Fred Gallo, Judith Swacks, Larry Nims, Asha Nahoma Clinton

Wilhelm Reich (orgone theory), Alexander Lowen (Bioenergetics)

(11) Electromagnetic Field (EMF) Lineage
The study of human, geophysical, astronomical, and artificial EMFs related fields: geopathic stress, dowsing, [Feng Shui]

(12) Quantum Physics Lineage
The study of the physics of non-material energy.

We could categorize those lineages that are concerned with healing along various lines; for instance, we may ask:

- Which part of the human energy anatomy is primarily addressed?
- What is the primary focus of the healing work (physical/emotional/mental/spiritual)?
- What is the nature of the healing energies employed?
- Is there a diagnostic component to the work? Who "diagnoses," and how is it done?

Appendix B

Reading Suggestions

We include the following reading suggestions as a service to those who wish to deepen their understanding of some of the topics touched upon in this book. The list is far from comprehensive and there are many other equally valuable publications.

Classics

- *Bhagavad-Gita,* translated by Prabhavananda & Christopher Isherwood (or others)
- *The Upanishads,* translated by Prabhavananda (or others)
- *Yoga,* by Vivekananda
- *Autobiography of a Yogi,* by Paramahansa Yogananda
- *Tao Te Ching*
- *The Tibetan Book of Living and Dying,* by Sogyal Rinpoche

Mind, Matter, and (Meta-) Physics

- *The Dreaming Universe*, by Fred Alan Wolf
- *Parallel Universes,* by Fred Alan Wolf
- *The Spiritual Universe,* by Fred Alan Wolf
- *The Eagle's Quest,* by Fred Alan Wolf
- *Mind into Matter,* by Fred Alan Wolf
- *The Holographic Universe,* by Michael Talbot
- *Mysticism and the New Physics,* by Michael Talbot
- *The Conscious Universe,* by Deepak Chopra
- *Infinite Mind,* by Valerie V. Hunt

- *The Numinous Universe,* by Daniel Liderbach
- *Quantum Mind,* by Arnold Mindell
- *Wholeness and the Implicate Order,* by David Bohm

The Human Energy Body

- *Aura Energy for Health, Healing & Balance,* by Joe H. Slate
- *How to See & Read the Aura,* by Ted Andrews
- *Hands of Light,* by Barbara A. Brennan
- *Man Visible and Invisible,* by C.W. Leadbeater
- *The Chakras,* by C.W. Leadbeater
- *Theories of the Chakras,* by Hiroshi Motoyama
- *Wheels of Light,* by Rosalyn L. Bruyere
- *Eastern Body, Western Mind,* by Anodea Judith
- *Book of Chakra Healing,* by Liz Simpson
- *Kundalini and the Chakras,* by Genevieve Lewis Paulson
- *A Chakra & Kudalini Workbook,* by John Mumford
- *The Awakening of Kundalini,* by Gopi Krishna
- *Kundalini Awakening,* by John Selby et al.
- *Energies of Transformation,* by Bonnie L. Greenwell
- *Balancing the Light Within,* by Linda Stein-Luthke & Martin F. Luthke

Vibrational Healing

- *The Healer's Manual,* by Ted Andrews
- *Quantum Healing,* by Deepak Chopra
- *Vibrational Medicine,* by Richard Gerber
- *Energy Medicine,* by James L. Oschman
- *Energy Medicine,* by Donna Eden
- *Anatomy of the Spirit,* by Caroline Myss

Reincarnation

- *Return from Tomorrow,* by George G. Ritchie with Elizabeth Sherrill
- *Life After Life,* by Raymond A. Moody
- *The Light Beyond,* by Raymond A. Moody
- *Many Lives, Many Masters,* by Brian L. Weiss
- *Reincarnation and Immortality,* by Rudolph Steiner
- *Reincarnation,* by Helen Wambach
- *Reliving Past Lives,* by Helen Wambach
- *The Case for Reincarnation,* by Joe Fisher
- *Children's Past Lives,* by Carol Bowman
- *Where Reincarnation and Biology Intersect,* by Ian Stevenson

Prayer, Affirmations, and Visualization

- *Prayer is Good Medicine,* by Larry Dossey
- *Reinventing Medicine,* by Larry Dossey
- *Healing Words,* by Larry Dossey
- *PrayWell,* by Walter L. Weston
- *You Can Heal Your Life,* by Louise Hay
- *Creative Visualization,* by Shakti Gawain
- *Affirmations and Thought Forms,* by Linda Stein-Luthke & Martin F. Luthke

Energy Psychology

- *Life Energy,* by John Diamond
- *Energy Tapping,* by Fred P. Gallo and Harry Vincenzi
- *Energy Diagnostic and Treatment Methods,* by Fred P. Gallo
- *Energy Psychology,* by Fred P. Gallo
- *Pranic Psychotherapy,* by Choa Kok Sui

- *You Can Heal Now,* by Tapas Fleming
- *Be Set Free Fast,* by Larry P. Nims
- *The Energy Psychology Desktop Companion,* by David Grudermeyer

Selected Web Sites

• www.energypsych.org : web site of the Association for Comprehensive Energy Psychology (ACEP); phone: 800-915-3606 x21; e-mail: acep@energypsych.org.

• selfhelpuniv.com: web site with information on Thought Field Therapy (TFT).

• www.emofree.com: Gary Craig's web site on the Emotional Freedom Techniques (EFT) with many links and resources (some free).

• www.wholistichealingresearch.com: web site with information on research on holistic healing, compiled by Daniel J. Benor, M.D.

• www.ttn.org: web site of the Transformation Training Network with many interesting links and definitions of various therapeutic approaches.

• www.energypsych.com: Dr. Fred Gallo's web site, with links.

• www.PsychInnovations.com: Informative web site on innovative psychotherapies, with links.

Appendix C

Other Books by the Authors

Expansion Publishing is offering the following titles by Linda Stein-Luthke and Martin F. Luthke, Ph.D.:

- ***Angels and Other Beings of Light:** **They are Here to Help You!** A Discourse from the Ascended Master St. Germain,* by Linda Stein-Luthke and Martin F. Luthke, ISBN 0-9656927-3-6, 84 pp., US $8.95. A channeled discourse on working with angels, Archangels, Ascended Masters, Twin Flame, soul mates, and other beings of Light; who they are; what their purpose is; how to contact them; how to experience your Higher Self; suggested readings.

- ***Balancing the Light Within.*** *A Discourse on Healing from the Ascended Master St. Germain,* by Linda Stein-Luthke and Martin F. Luthke, ISBN 0-9656927-0-1, 54 pp., US $5.00. A channeled discourse on light vibrations, tools of awareness, chakras, healing of self and others with metaphysical means; suggested readings.

- ***Affirmations and Thought Forms:** **You Can Change Your Mind!** A Discourse from the Ascended Master St. Germain,* by Linda Stein-Luthke and Martin F. Luthke, ISBN 0-9656927-1-X, 48 pp., US $5.00. A channeled discourse on the use of affirmations and the power of thought forms and how to use both for healing purposes, with emphasis on self-empowerment and self-awareness; suggested readings.

• ***Riding the Tide of Change*: Preparing for Personal & Planetary Transformation,** by Martin F. Luthke, ISBN 0-9656927-2-8, 108 pp., US $9.95. A metaphysical book on Earth changes with an emphasis on releasing fears, healing self and understanding our role as co-creators during this time of transformation; suggested readings. (Several of the chapters from *Riding the Tide of Change* have been revised and incorporated in *Beyond Psychotherapy*; thus, if you have read the latter, you may not wish to buy the former.)

• ***Beyond Psychotherapy*: Introduction to Psychoenergetic Healing,** by Martin F. Luthke and Linda Stein-Luthke, ISBN 0-9656927-4-4, 228 pp., US $19.95.

How to Order Books

• **For more information**: For more information, excerpts, and secure on-line orders, please visit ***www.u-r-light.com***. You may e-mail any inquiries to ***expansion@u-r-light.com***. Please contact us for overseas orders or quantity discounts.

• **On-line orders**: Please visit http://***www.u-r-light.com***.

• **Mail-in orders**: Please send your order -- including your e-mail address, if available -- to: Expansion Publishing, P.O. Box 516, Chagrin Falls, OH 44022, USA. Shipping: Please add $2.00 for orders totaling up to $10 and $4.00 for orders over $10. US-checks or money orders.

• **Bookstores**: All titles are also available through your local bookstore. However, you may need to special-order them.

• **Phone orders**: Please call **Book Clearing House** (800-356-9315) for 24-hour credit card orders.